Industry's Voice in Health Policy

WITH CONTRIBUTIONS BY

George N. Bates, M.D.
Owens–Illinois, Inc.

W. Gordon Binns, Jr.
General Motors Corporation

John Brown
Genesco, Inc.

Harry P. Cain, Jr.
American Health Planning Association

Irvine H. Dearnley
Citibank

H. Peter deLisser
The Executive Health Examiners Group

Henry A. DiPrete
John Hancock Mutual Life Insurance
Company

Paul W. Earle
The Voluntary Effort

Richard H. Egdahl, M.D.
Boston University Center for Industry
and Health Care

Paul M. Ellwood, Jr., M.D.
InterStudy

Richard E. Emrick
Mead Corporation

Jonathan E. Fielding, M.D.
Commonwealth of Massachusetts

Max W. Fine
Committee for National Health
Insurance

Frank E. Finkenberg
George B. Buck Consulting Actuaries,
Inc.

Scott Fleming
Kaiser Foundation Health Plan, Inc.

Cramer M. Gilmore, II
International Brotherhood of the
Teamsters Union

Willis B. Goldbeck
Washington Business Group on Health

Clark C. Havighurst, J.D.
Duke University, American Enterprise
Institute, and Federal Trade Commission

Lawrence C. Horowitz, M.D.
Senate Subcommittee on Health and
Scientific Research

Samuel H. Howard
Hospital Affiliates International, Inc.

Ronald A. Hurst
Caterpillar Tractor Company

Stanley B. Jones
Institute of Medicine

Ronald H. Kilgren
Ford Motor Company

H. Peter Kneen, Jr.
IBM Corporation

Joseph G. Kozlowski
TRW, Inc.

Philip R. Lescohier
William M. Mercer, Inc.

J. Michael McGinnis, M.D.
Department of Health, Education, and
Welfare

Judith K. Miller
National Health Policy Forum

Kenneth J. Morrissey
FMC Corporation

Joseph N. Onek
The White House

Jan Peter Ozga
U.S. Chamber of Commerce

John J. Salmon
U.S. House of Representatives

Bert Seidman
AFL–CIO

Nila A. Vehar
Koppers Company, Inc.

Howard R. Veit
Office of Health Maintenance
Organizations

John R. Virts, Ph.D.
Eli Lilly and Company

Kenneth W. White
Health Insurance Institute

Daniel I. Zwick
American Hospital Association

INDUSTRY AND HEALTH CARE 7

Industry's Voice in Health Policy

EDITED BY
Richard H. Egdahl
Diana Chapman Walsh

GUEST EDITOR
Willis B. Goldbeck

 Springer-Verlag   New York

Springer Series on Industry and Health Care
Richard H. Egdahl, M.D., Ph.D.
Diana Chapman Walsh, M.S.
Center for Industry and Health Care
Boston University Health Policy Institute
53 Bay State Road
Boston, Massachusetts 02215

Springer-Verlag New York Inc.
175 Fifth Avenue
New York, New York 10010

Library of Congress Cataloging in Publication Data
Main entry under title:

Industry's voice in health policy.

    (Springer series on industry and health care; 7)
    Based on the Washington Business Group on Health's 1978 annual meeting.
    Includes index.
    1. Medical policy—United States—Congresses. 2. Medical policy—United
States—Business community participation—Congresses. I. Egdahl, Richard H.
II. Walsh, Diana Chapman. III. Washington Business Group on Health.
RA395.A3I493   338.4'7'36210973   79-16023

The use of general descriptive names, trade names, trademarks, etc. in this publication,
even if the former are not especially identified, is not to be taken as a sign that such
names, as understood by the Trade Marks and Merchandise Marks Act, may accordingly
be used freely by anyone.

Printed in the United States of America

9 8 7 6 5 4 3 2 1

ISBN 0-387-90429-8 Springer-Verlag New York Heidelberg Berlin
ISBN 3-540-90429-8 Springer-Verlag Berlin Heidelberg New York

Preface

It is a pleasure to introduce this special volume of the Industry and Health Care Series. It is special for the best of reasons: it is primarily written by industry representatives. Using the Washington Business Group on Health 1978 Annual Meeting as its starting point, this volume captures the feelings, concerns, and experience of many who are leading industry's increasingly significant presence in health policy and economics.

While many of the largest companies achieve more sophisticated levels of involvement, the fact remains that most companies of all sizes and especially the smaller businesses either will not or cannot devote the time or resources to become active participants. We hope this volume will help demonstrate the value of even one person's commitment.

Although our organizational focus is Washington, the WBGH recognizes that, in the long run, the quality and cost of the health care most Americans receive will be—and should be—determined at the local level. To let this happen without industry involvement would represent an abdication of both responsibility and opportunity.

Fortunately, we see a growth of industry involvement, growth not just in terms of numbers but also in terms of the scope of activities.

- Recognizing that the key to changing provider behavior is to change the economic incentives, emanating from the major payers, employers are subjecting their employee benefit plans to the most complete scrutiny in many years.

- Corporate officers are being trained to assume new, more aggressive and businesslike roles on hospital boards.
- Government and industry are increasingly aware of their common interests, and through such programs as health planning and HMO development they are working more cooperatively than ever before.
- There is growing interest in shifting the orientation of industrial medicine and health benefits away from acute care and toward prevention.

In the next few years, with or without increased government health regulation, we predict a veritable boom in industry involvement in health care.

- Claims monitoring and control will enter a new era of sophistication and rigor with a basic philosophy that these new controls will actually enhance the quality of the employee's health and health benefits.
- Employers will increasingly aggregate their health care efforts into community-level coalitions. Cost containment will dominate the agenda but only for the first few years, after which access and quality will return as the primary policy issues.
- Medical technology, health education, and mental well-being will become major new areas of industry concern.

Industry is not the answer to our nation's health care financing and delivery problem, but industry does hold several of the critical keys necessary to unlock the current system and open it for responsible change.

The WBGH is very pleased to have the opportunity to continue our growing relationship with Dick Egdahl and Diana Walsh of the Boston University Center for Industry and Health Care and to participate in this series. Through these cooperative efforts, we hope industry will gain an increased appreciation for its role in health policy, a role we feel to be essential if our health system is to improve for the benefit of all.

Washington, March 1979   Willis B. Goldbeck
                                                                  Guest Editor

Preface

This seventh issue of the Industry and Health Care Series derives from an evolving collaboration between the Center for Industry and Health Care of Boston University and the Washington Business Group on Health. As must any successful relationship, this collaboration enables two complementary organizations to reinforce one another in ways that are mutually beneficial and yet respectful of the independent integrity of each.

The Center for Industry and Health Care emerged in early 1977 as a separate entity within the Boston University Health Policy Institute. Created to study the organization, financing, and delivery of health services to employees in private industry and to work with corporations and unions on their cost containment strategies, the Center's originating hypothesis was that private industry can be a key force in the national effort to stabilize health care costs while preserving the good features of the existing delivery system. Since its genesis the Center has endeavored, through conferences, consultations, and publications, to develop an identity and a distinct competence that has meaning to its constituency.

The quarterly Industry and Health Care Series is both product and instrument of the commitment to become as pragmatic and realistic a resource as possible. Individual volumes of the series now build on consultations with industry and on meetings convened to explore with management and labor specific concerns that they bring to our attention. Examples are the self-insurance option, probed in the spring issue of the series, and the special health problems of women workers, to be the focus of next winter's monograph. Now in its second year, the series has been adapted in various ways to incorporate readers' suggestions; with each successive issue, we have come to feel more surefooted on what was originally not the most familiar terrain.

While all of this was taking shape, the Washington Business Group on Health, which antedates the Center by two and a half years, had established itself in Washington as a strong, steady, and credible source of information on corporate health programs and on the perspective on health policy issues of major private purchaser of care. The information collected by the WBGH had not previously been available to the formulators of public policy in health. The WBGH has developed an extraordinary capacity for rapid, focused, and timely responses to the informational needs of Congress, the executive branch, the states, and even community level organizations. Bill Goldbeck and his staff have become indispensible to corporate medical and benefits directors interested in cost containment in health, and indeed to some chief executives and corporate boards now sensitized to the urgency of the cost problem in health.

In the process of emerging, the two groups have interacted easily and naturally—the Washington Business Group on Health, with an extensive network of corporate and government contacts and detailed knowledge of industrial health programming, the Center for Industry and Health Care, with expertise in alternative delivery systems, targeted educational programs in health planning and resource allocation and the somewhat greater detachment and time for reflection possible in academia. For our part, the close association with the members and staff of the WBGH has been a major wellspring of creativity and strength.

Within the context of this relationship, it seemed a logical next step in the evolution of the Industry and Health Care Series to devote one issue each year to the annual meeting of the WBGH, which represents a synthesis and stock-taking of corporate perspectives on the year's health policy developments. With the help of Bill Goldbeck and his staff, we were able at the 1978 meeting to enlist some key participants who agreed to take time, in weeks following the meeting, to prepare the commentaries that appear in this book. Meanwhile, Anthony J. Mahler and Janet K. Marantz did a yeomanly job of extracting, summarizing, and editing the transcription of the meeting, and Antonette Doherty kept track of it all.

As the commentaries flowed into our office and we saw the added dimensions they were bringing to the meeting itself we became progressively more enthusiastic about the book. It strongly conveys the message that although the "private sector" does not speak with one voice on matters of health policy, it *is* now speaking with a collection of voices that are well-informed and concerned, sometimes perplexed or combative, but invariably thoughtful and provocative. All of the contributors to the book have our thanks for making this an unusual, useful, and we think potentially influential issue of the series.

Boston, March 1979   Richard H. Egdahl

Diana Chapman Walsh

Contents

INTRODUCTION

I

A Challenge to Industry

Willis B. Goldbeck

I spend a lot of my life traveling over the country talking to groups about industry: trying to represent industry's concerns, presenting the accomplishments of the last few years, and providing other segments of our society with some comprehension of what this funny thing called "industry health care" is all about. I would like to share with you a few of my concerns and thoughts about the issues I have encountered. I have picked ten points to lay before you, hoping that they will stimulate our discussions during this conference.

Industry's Evolving Role As Questioning Purchaser of Health Care

The first point to stress is that the involvement of industry in health care has been evolving over the last few years, coming from what I can only characterize as a passive stance, up through an attentiveness to the government's health policies, and finally to increasing self-examination. Industry now examines what it is doing in health care and why, and what its values are. This has led to some action programs and innovations that are attracting increased attention, including attention from government . . . sort of a turnaround. Industry today stands on the verge of becoming a true consumer of health care—a role in which some businesspeople may not feel overly comfortable, but which has tremendous economic implications for our country because of the massive amount of money involved.

Providers and governments have difficulty implementing true cost containment programs because such programs require a change in providers' incentives. Industry, though, can help. It is certainly not easy for companies to make dramatic changes in reimbursement systems and, particularly, in how much individuals might end up paying personally. Nonetheless, there remain tremendous numbers of things you can do in the design of the benefits you provide and in whom you choose to pay. There are many, many things you can do as you manage the data as well as the dollars of your system. To fail to do so is to fail to take advantage of the one opportunity left with the private sector to seize the reins of the health care system.

It is very important to recognize that you can purchase health care in precisely the way you purchase any other product, and if that disturbs some of the providers, so be it. There is no reason why the purchase of any product should be a decision devoid of an interest in quality or in waste. Quality need not get mired down in the waste issue. Every hospital in the United States does not need to exist as it currently is. Indeed, not all of them need to exist, period. If industry is serious about cost containment and is serious about quality, you must recognize what the trade-offs are, what tough policy and value decisions need to be made, and where economic leverage must be brought to bear. If not, then go ahead and pay for thousands of empty beds in your community, pay for false and unnecessary claims, pay for lots of unnecessary surgery, acquiesce to providers, employees, or dependents who equate unthinking demand with need. However, remember that you are using your stockholders' money, your employees' money, and your profits to pay for health care that is not really needed. That's really what it comes down to, and in this era of limited resources none of us can afford that kind of waste.

Closing "Gaps" in the System: An Agenda We Cannot Ignore

My second point is that concern for costs, be it by industry or government or any other segment of society, cannot be allowed to obscure the very real human needs out there that must be addressed. This underlies a great deal of the pressure for increased government intervention. Basically, industry and the private sector have a choice: ignore those needs or try to close as many of the gaps as possible. Both choices are very expensive, but there is a critical economic reason why, I would suggest, closing the gaps is the wiser approach. Poverty is by far the most expensive waste in the United States today, and there are millions of people who need health services that they are not getting and cannot get. Issues such as the waiting period for benefits to begin, how to deal with people who are laid off, how to deal with part-time and temporary employees—these are examples of what are often called in testimony "cracks in the system." Such cracks in the system are what drive various government agencies and members of Congress and its committees to take action if the private sector demonstrates either an unwillingness or an inability to close them. I say that fully cognizant of the fact that closing any of those gaps costs a lot of money. The questions that we all must face in the next year or two are, Who is it better to have close those gaps? and What are the long-term costs?

From Headquarters to the Hinterlands

The third point I would like to make is that there is a crying need for increased communication from the corporate headquarters to the local level in virtually all companies, even in the most dynamic. I still, as I travel around the country, find benefits managers, division personnel people, plant managers and so on who either say, "We have no responsibility for health; that's handled at headquarters," or they have never had any communication to give them reason or encouragement to become involved in health issues. Rarely are there any direct incentives for local people to spend the time, energy, and corporate resources that such involvement would require.

In a great many communities there are no corporate headquarters, and so it is going to be very important how local-level people in your companies conduct themselves in the next few years. They are the ones who have to face the planning issues, the HMO issues, the interaction with local government on local health issues. This is what is really going to determine whether industry and health care interact through small leadership groups, such as we have here today, or whether a nationwide movement will effect dramatic change.

I would suggest one simple step: make every local element of your company responsible for health even if, in fact, they are not responsible for actual financial allocations. They need to be made responsible to you for their health care costs as a stimulus for becoming involved in the system or at least learning about it at the local level. Your local people have a job to do. Top management of major corporations needs to recognize that at the local level it may be a department store and not you that is the largest employer, and that the department store, with a little stimulus from your company, may in fact be best situated to get action and provide leadership at that local level.

Another local endeavor that definitely needs assistance is the health care activity of local chambers of commerce. Most do not have any health committee, and the vast majority of those that do have a provider as chairperson. Many industry people around the country say, "That committee is useless to us for that very reason." I would like to see them vote the provider out of the chairmanship and vote one of themselves in. These local chambers can be very effective focal points of industry activity.

The Next Step: Local Coalitions

My fourth point is that coalitions of businesses at the local level must be the next step in the evolutionary process of industrial involvement in health care. These need not be viewed as anticompetitive. There is no reason in the world why all the auto companies or all the oil companies or all of any other industry segment can't agree to work together in a given town on health policy issues, even though they may be competing like blazes on their own product lines. Someone must take the lead. In setting up local health consortia, don't wait for university groups and others to come to you and suggest that you get together. Go to them. It will be cheaper in the long run, and you will be in charge.

Industry must also make a special effort to bring small business into the picture. This is not at all a charity suggestion. The small business issue is gaining increased political significance. When we meet with the White House or with congressional groups now, we are consistently asked, "What will this mean to small business?" This question was not even raised two years ago, and no high-visibility organization like the WBGH exists for small businesses to turn to. To the extent you can help in that area, you will be performing a major service for every part of industry in the United States.

Industry's Obligations to the Voluntary Effort

My fifth point concerns the Voluntary Effort. The central issue with the VE is simply that it is there, and whether or not there is another legislative program next year, industry has a serious responsibility to make the VE work.

I certainly do not mean to be coopted by the VE. In fact, it is essential that industry work to bring accountability to it. No statistic that the VE puts out should be accepted by you just because they put it out. It should be accepted by you only if you have good, sound reasons to believe it. VE can be a cartel, as it has been described, or it can be made accountable. Industry can make the difference.

During the latter day stages of the debate in Congress on cost containment bills when it looked fairly certain that no bill was going to pass, providers in communities all over the United States began to get complacent. I have talked with a dozen hospital associations and numerous medical groups in the last six months, and, almost to a person, they talked about how they had "won" on the cost containment legislative issue, and a lot of them thought they had "won" with our help. In fact, they probably did, with some of our help. But if that degree of complacency is allowed to continue at the local level, and if industry doesn't make the provider groups recognize fully that there won't be any "victory" two years from now if the VE fails, then we are asking for whatever we get in terms of cost escalation and government regulation. A significant amount of the onus is on us.

Where Government Fits

My sixth point is that we will need in the next two years a dramatic growth in the involvement of industry in health care at the state and local government level because they are the two major pressure areas for state and federal intervention. We all know how difficult it is to take any action with benefit plans designed as they are, with the lack of competition in health services, and with the growth of state and federal regulation that decreases the arena over which you apparently have any control. However, it is interesting to note that the state that probably has the largest amount of health regulation, Minnesota, also has the largest amount of health competition in the private sector. Apparently, there are ways to blend the two. They are not absolutely antithetical, and examples of making them work together deserve very careful scrutiny.

The seventh point refers to, putting it bluntly, who gets the dirty end of the stick in terms of health care costs if the system is to shrink. There is no single answer, of course, but it is clear that industry will get a disproportionate share of the stick if it fails to manage its resource allocations and its expenditures a lot better than it has in the past. At the same time, it cannot do these things responsibly if it pushes costs off on the poorer segments of the population. I find it a basic inconsistency that industry on the one hand says, "Leave all these groups to the government . . . the poor, and the near-poor, and particularly the varied segments of society that are difficult and expensive for us to

handle," but then they add "But we also do not want any more government involvement in health care." I would suggest that in our
discussions, and particularly as we complain about things that government is doing, that we do not talk in global terms. Rather, let us try
to find out those segments of regulations that have no basis in fact, that
have no logical, real reason to have come into being, and focus on
trying to get them stricken from the books. This is better than a broad
diatribe against government.

A Time for Accountability

The eighth point concerns accountability. I question whether most
companies feel they have a say in or feel very positive about the
insurance industry's public relations campaign. I don't know whether
it's a good idea or a bad idea, but I do know that any such megadollar
endeavors need a very high degree of input from industry, preferably
not after they are implemented. For the future, industry needs to work
with the carriers to make sure that a segment of the public relations
effort evolves into concrete programs at the local level. The next ad
shouldn't just dramatize the cost problem, but instead can say what the
carriers and industry have done together in some town to actually
achieve both quality health care and cost containment.

It is also time that we demanded a great deal more accountability
from the providers that industry is paying. And, we must recognize that
it is possible to require more self-responsibility of your employees, or at
least not equate their demand for something with an actual need for it. I
find it disturbing to be told by corporate people in a meeting on
nutrition issues, "If the employees ask to have sugar candy in the
vending machines, we have to put it there." I doubt if the response
would be the same if they asked for alcohol. Where is the cut-off point?
I don't know, but we have to look for it.

It is also possible to make second surgical opinion programs mandatory. If you are paying the benefits and if you already require a great
many things of your employees in the health care area—for instance, an
entry level physical or periodical physicals—then you can also require
other things. If you think second surgical opinions are worth experimenting with, I can assure you that they are not worth experimenting
with on a one percent voluntary utilization.

Values, Decision Criteria, and Definitional Dilemmas

Let me bring up, then, my ninth point. New values underlie our
capacity and willingness to make changes in reimbursement systems
and to deal with government correctly and positively, but they are not

always well thought out. The broad question is, What is appropriate in terms of health care delivery?, and our answers are changing. People are now beginning to question the appropriateness of intensive care, for instance. A few studies have shown that cardiac patients and accident victims appear to do at least as well and, in some cases, better when treated at home than when wired up on the apparatus in the hospital.

Mental well-being is another area where what we frequently hear are value judgments: "Well, we did a program ten years ago that was overutilized, so we don't want to do one now." That is not the way you would make a decision on any other facet of your business, and that is not the way we should make decisions in the mental well-being arena from now on. The studies of the Kaiser system, and others, have indicated that an incredible number of office visits are by people who are physically well but worried, and industry is paying the bill for them.

The value question is whether one wants to treat health as an investment, not just a benefit, and I think we need more understanding of the relations among health care costs, disability, retraining, reemployment costs, absenteeism, and productivity. We also need, it seems to me, to recognize that the term *employee benefits* may be a misnomer. You insure a great many more dependents and you pay a great deal more for dependents', claims than you do for employees; yet the vast majority of all cost containment strategies focus strictly on the employee. Somehow or other, the employee benefit process must grasp much more clearly the life style of the dependent who may be the high utilizer of medical benefits.

Business Leadership in Community Programs: Public Health and School Health

My last point concerns businesspeople in the role of community leaders, as a great many of you are. Many community leaders interact with the health care system, but for some reason choose to do so not as businesspeople but as charity-givers. There are many communities in the United States where the public health facilities, for instance, could benefit tremendously from some management assistance, from some advice, even from some understanding of the needs of local employers. The communication level is low, low, low, but it is exciting to see examples of where people have gotten together. Dick Martin of Goodyear, for example, has spent a lot of time with the public health people in Akron, Ohio, and feels that both the company and the community have benefited fantastically.

I would also emphasize health education in the schools, which is usually absent. Many of you or your spouses are on school boards or various PTA committees, yet very rarely do we see an interaction between all the knowledge you have accumulated about health care and school health education. There are over 16,000 school districts in the United States, the vast majority of which do not have one hour of health education in their entire twelve-year curriculum. How are we supposed to get the next generation to understand our bodies, ourselves, and the health care system out of that kind of education background? It won't happen, and neither will cost containment. I have heard numerous corporate officers say, "The school system is supposed to take care of it." Fine. But, if it isn't doing it, it doesn't help to keep saying it's supposed to unless we make it do so and make it accountable for doing so.

Let me close by stressing two words: credibility and integrity. They relate to you as a human resource for the government, for providers, for other industries. You are the cream of the crop—whether you like the designation or not, you are stuck with it. You do know more about health care than most other people in industry, and it is incumbent on you to put that knowledge to use. There is no reason to acquiesce to the demands of government or the demands of the providers or the demands of labor. That should be past history for industry in health care. But to resist brings with it the responsibility to exercise the leadership of which you are clearly capable. It is our pleasure to work with you in this effort.

Question Period

Q.: Could you elaborate on your point about the greater value of home care over hospital care in some cases?

Mr. Goldbeck: There is a reconsideration abroad in the land as to how much people need and respond physiologically and psychologically to being wired up to vast numbers of machines, to awakening in a hospital atmosphere, and so on. This is not to imply that there is anything inherently wrong or improper being done by those institutions. Rather, it is a question of degrees and proper judgments by medical authorities as to who can go home and convalesce in a more pleasant setting. The whole hospice concept recognizes the value of one's family and natural surroundings as a part of the medical intervention. Also, there is a problem with infection in hospitals, and a great many people receive iatrogenic, in other words, unintended, "provider-caused" diseases and injuries.

Q.: On the subject of the school setting for education and nutrition, I have two questions. First, when my kids tell me what they're learning I have been shocked at how out-of-date and erroneous the material in their health programs is. Is there any chance that this group could take a look itself without going through HEW at the curricula that are available and see if they could be improved? Second, is there a possibility that you could take a look at whether school feeding programs are being used as a vehicle for educating kids in good nutritional habits?

Mr. Goldbeck: Those are two good points indeed. On the question of taking a look at curricula, we have begun to do so slightly. I'm on a couple of the steering committees for both government and private school health education programs that are being conducted right now. We are trying to get a handle on what's in these programs. It is a very difficult issue and, very frankly, one of the big problems is local church groups that intervene very strenuously in school health curricula. There is an unfortunate identification of school health education with sex education.

On the question of food services, there is growing concern with that because so much of the food in school lunch programs ends up in the waste basket instead of in the kids. Whether that is a healthy result or not remains to be seen, depending on where that food comes from. One of the new approaches that has been used is the fast food concept of school feeding which, indeed, does get the kids to eat, and apparently, the dietitians are able to package those foods so that they have a highly nutritious content. But this approach tends to mask the nutrition issue, and it may very well be missing a good opportunity to bring kids along to understanding more about nutrition, health education, and their bodies in general.

Kenneth Morrissey, FMC Corporation: As a member of an HSA in the Chicago area, I would recommend a simple way for everyone to get involved in local health planning. Just get hold of your HSA's annual implementation plan and look it over, and you can easily get involved in health planning in your community. The plan is easily available— look at it and see what they have in there for you and for your community.

Mr. Goldbeck: I certainly endorse that. As a footnote, I would add that those of you with facilities located in Los Angeles should get involved in the new HSA being started in that area. It's a very large HSA, and it's located in one of the areas where there's more waste than anywhere else in the country. There was no industry involvement in that area's first HSA, which recently failed, so by all means, get involved out there if you possibly can.

Peter deLisser, Executive Health Examiners: In your travels, does the issue of privacy come up in relation to cost containment?

Mr. Goldbeck: Yes, it does. Privacy and confidentiality are issues that many benefits people face regularly. About all one can say generally about them is that most companies don't really want to delve into their employee records in an overly invasionary fashion, and most never do so. Real violations seem to come to the fore pretty fast and pretty loudly. I think it is quite possible to do the bulk of cost containment without any violation of anybody's privacy.

James Tobin, Becton-Dickenson: Another resource that corporations can use to influence the health care system is their contributions budget. Corporations traditionally give a lot of money to hospitals for construction, but perhaps they should require certificates of need, provide incentives for restructuring the health care system, and provide contributions to phase out unneeded beds.

Mr. Goldbeck: That's a valid point, and it's the kind of issue we are going to be facing in the next few years. Many of the upcoming issues are not quality-of-care, but purely and simply economic. The health system and the health of Americans will be better for industry's participation.

COMMENTARY

Nila A. Vehar, Staff Coordinator, Government Affairs, Koppers Company, Inc.

Mr. Goldbeck has challenged all of industry to accept the responsibility for leadership as this nation prepares to develop a national health policy that will, in one way or another, impact all Americans. His suggestions run the gamut from increasing business participation in local health planning to translating new social values—the issues of dying, mental well-being, and health education—into quality programs. The call for business to enter this policy arena is welcome, but let's not lose sight of some questions along the way.

How do we balance the tensions between human needs and existing social facts? Can we properly deal with the overlapping of public authority and private interests? How does public policy balance costs against perceived benefits? Who are the custodians of the American people? And, for this particular issue, what level of health care do we intend to provide for what segments of society?

As business increases its participation in public policymaking, it will face these and other questions. The responsibility of business and other institutions is to leave preconceived notions at the doorstep and enter the public debate with the intention of breaking down barriers between traditional adversary groups. Recognition, respect, and understanding of opposing viewpoints are the prerequisites for a purposeful dialogue on meeting the real needs of society. The desire to grow beyond our own limitations will, I think, help in the crucial debate on health policy.

We all feel some concern over the rapid growth of government intervention into what was previously seen as a private sector responsibility. Many of us believe that government is best when it governs least, or, stated another way, that the government is supposed to keep hands off private interests unless the public interest clearly justifies intervention. Sometimes it helps to reflect on the past so that we can understand the present and adapt to future change. A hundred years ago, the notion of compulsory education was a radical idea; fire protection, water treatment, and sewage disposal were not considered government responsibilities; there were no pure food and drug laws; and there were no safety, health, or environmental laws. I am not suggesting that all government intervention solves all society's problems, nor that it always equals the expectations of the public. But, it is clear that when the government perceives an inability on the part of private institutions to satisfy societal needs, it will attempt to mandate solutions.

The escalation of interest in a national health policy stems, in part, from a widespread belief that quality health care is a matter of right. The public has challenged our political system to respond to that belief. What happens during the next decade will depend on many economic and political pressures, but the quality of the decision will rest on the ability of various institutions to seek the truth and develop support for a policy that satisfies the real needs of our society.

Through participation and self-analysis, we can help government develop a national health policy that strengthens existing private mechanisms, eliminates waste, and contains costs, and one that finds ways for providing health education, protection, and quality care for those who do not have access to them. Congress is looking for advice, ideas, and cooperation from business and other segments of society as it proceeds to balance interests on this crucial issue. We have the experience, the talent, and the imagination, so let's accept the challenge.

COMMENTARY

George N. Bates, M.D., Medical Director, Owens-Illinois, Inc.

Industry pays a large portion of the nation's health care bill, and it is well for Mr. Goldbeck to comment that business must come to view itself as a consumer as well as a producer—insisting on a consumer's right to know the product and to understand and react to its sale and delivery.

Mr. Goldbeck believes that exercising such an option might well alter the incentives currently urging on the providers of health care. Yet, he also feels that if there are gaps in the perceived response to health care needs, industry must address them even though this could be cost stimulating. Although there are voices railing against any further increases in health care because of its cost, most of us would prefer to satisfy any legitimate health care needs. Priorities thus need both assignment and alignment, and reasonable people should be able to develop reasonable alternatives to accomplish this goal.

If industry has a legitimate interest in controlling the cost of health care while improving its delivery, then the local operations of big business need to accept responsibility for influence in their communities. Each component of local interest may well be very important, and that overworked word and underworked concept—*communication*—must be understood and then employed. An aggregation of businesses, large and small, should exert its influence appropriately. This aggregation must study the issues and espouse the cause of controlling health care costs, never diluting its influence in spurious or poorly understood positions.

The Voluntary Effort currently appears to have little support from industry for several reasons, not the least of which is business's lack of a prior demonstration of voluntarism on its own part. But industry should engender and then deliver support. The sooner accountability is insisted upon from the VE, the sooner this effort will be viable and the sooner there will be a leveling effect on cost. Every legitimate containment opportunity should be grasped, but not at the expense of rationing quality health care. The VE is a project well worth encouraging.

Mr. Goldbeck agrees with this position but does not seem very optimistic about the success of the VE. From the standpoint of past experience, his reaction may well be justified. But the VE currently does enjoy success, and it needs support even though some of us wonder about its vitality.

Industry's involvement, locally and at the state level, must mature or we will continue to face expanding costs. Accountability is the handle. Too much time has been spent on defining the problem and too little on its solution. We are all aware of this, but Mr. Goldbeck is wise to reiterate it. Lamenting over the problem will be nonproductive while, as Mr. Goldbeck would have us believe, there are management methods currently at our disposal that could make a difference. We need policies and programs.

The members of the WBGH now have a better comprehension

of cost containment, and with this comes an increased responsibility to influence the thinking of hospital boards and local public health boards. Schools must be made responsive and accountable on their health education curricula. Providers will simply have to be shown that the milieu of their practices has undergone a transformation.

It has been demonstrated repeatedly, but it must be said again that costs have to be contained by such actions as the use of outpatient services in lieu of inpatient services where appropriate, shorter length of inpatient stay, preadmission testing, weekend laboratory activities, alternative forms of health care delivery, and many, many more. Even more helpful would be a reduction in the demand for very expensive health care services, but this may be difficult to accomplish in the face of demand. But, we do, after all, have an obligation to care for ourselves. It is time we took this obligation seriously and stopped being burdensome to one another.

GOVERNMENT
PERSPECTIVES

II

President Carter's Principles for Health Care Cost Containment and National Health Insurance

Joseph N. Onek

The Carter White House has two major concerns regarding health care: cost containment and national health insurance. Let me describe our initiatives in each of these areas.

The problem of cost containment from the government's point of view is most obviously reflected in the budgetary increases for Medicare and Medicaid. In a few years these programs have grown from 4.3 percent of the federal budget to 12.7 percent. Taxpayers are painfully aware that the payroll tax for Medicare, which began at 0.7 percent, is now 2.1 percent. In addition, a wide variety of federal, state, and local taxes support the Medicaid program. Much of the increase in the cost of these programs is due to health care cost inflation, which has exceeded 15 percent per year.

Health care costs have also had a significant impact on general inflation. They appear in the Consumer Price Index not only under that little rubric called "health care," but throughout the economy because corporations are paying higher health insurance costs and passing them on through higher prices. Rising health care costs have thus had a dramatic impact both on our tax burden and on general inflation.

Ironically, this is happening just as many experts are beginning to argue that better health depends less on medical care than on other factors. For example, the leading cause of death among Americans under forty is automobile accidents. The second leading cause of death among white teenagers is suicide, and among black teenagers, homicide. So for the young, our most crucial health problems are not traditionally medical, and our greatest efforts have to be in other directions.

The second leading cause of death among all Americans is cancer, and some estimate that about 90 percent of cancers are environmentally caused. I am using *environmentally* here in the broadest sense to include behavioral factors, such as smoking and dietary habits, as well as air and water pollution. Here, too, we need to make inroads, and we're not going to make them through traditional medical care. But other efforts require both manpower and money, and we can not make them unless we bring medical costs under control.

Controlling health care costs is not a new idea. When we came into office, there was a proposal pending from the Ford administration to put a 7.5 percent ceiling on Medicare and Medicaid expenditures. We did not follow this approach for two reasons. First, if you only cap Medicare and Medicaid, you are inducing providers to discriminate against the beneficiaries of these programs. Second, we were assured by private insurance companies, among others, that providers would try to recoup the lost income by imposing greater expenses on everyone else. So we believe that the only sensible approach is an across-the-board cost containment effort.

Our proposal was to put a ceiling on hospital revenue from any and all sources. As you know, this proposal did not get through Congress in the past session, in part because of lack of support from the business community. We will reintroduce hospital cost controls in the next year, and I hope that business will consider supporting them. There is a natural reluctance to support a program that looks on its surface like mandatory price controls of the kind that both business and the President have opposed. But there are tremendous differences between the hospital industry and other industries—differences that make the term *price control* inapplicable.

First, hospital use is not a free market decision. Most patients choose neither the hospital they go to nor the services they receive. These choices are made by their physicians. Second, none of the usual incentives for efficiency exist because 93 percent of all hospital bills are paid by third parties. Finally, it is even inaccurate to talk about "prices" in a situation where programs such as Blue Cross and Medicare pay on a cost-reimbursement basis. Business has begun to realize that the health care sector is different. For example, the business community has not only supported but has actively participated in health planning and certificate of need programs, programs that it would probably not support elsewhere in the economy.

What we are trying to do for government, and what I'm sure you are trying to do for industry, is to become prudent buyers. We want something more like a contract than an open-ended, limitless reimbursement system. Most people in the field agree that we have to move toward a prospective reimbursement system; our cost containment program is a step in that direction.

We are also pursuing other nonregulatory approaches to dealing with health care cost inflation. We are trying to foster competition through alternative delivery systems such as HMOs. In Minneapolis–St. Paul, for example, there has been tremendous support by business for HMOs, and there seems to be real competition acting to reduce medical care costs. HMOs need two things to get off the ground: they need capital and they need effective managerial leadership. The government can provide capital, but it cannot provide entrepreneurial and managerial skill. Only one institution in our society can provide that and it is the business community.

And, of course, prevention efforts can also help reduce total costs. Hypertensive screening programs, alcohol programs, physical fitness programs—in these and other ways, the business community can contribute and is contributing. Clearly, regulation is not the only solution.

The second item on President Carter's agenda is the closely related issue of NHI. Our country needs NHI because some 19 million Americans still have no public or private health insurance, and an estimated 85 million have no protection from catastrophic medical costs. Neither problem exists in most other developed countries, and they really should not exist here.

Most of the countries in Western Europe have some form of NHI program, although the programs differ widely. They range from the British model of government-employed, salaried physicians to the German program, which consists of several thousand private insurance organizations. But, no matter what the form or structure of the program, there is nobody in those countries who cannot afford to go to a doctor for basic needs, and nobody who's going to be devastated by large medical bills. The President is supporting an NHI program for these reasons, as well as because he feels that it can provide greater opportunities to control costs.

As you know, the President issued ten principles on NHI last summer, focusing on the two concerns of access and inflation. Let me summarize some of the principles briefly.

The President's first principle is that given present budgetary restraints, there will be no new expenditures until fiscal 1983. Second, when expenditures are made they will be phased in gradually. And third, we must allow future administrations the discretion to delay or suspend NHI or take other action in light of then-current economic conditions.

In addition to the very strong commitment against making NHI an inflationary program, two other features of the President's principles deserve emphasis. First, the President made it clear that NHI was not to be a totally government-run program. Financing would be through both tax revenues and employer-employee contributions of the type that now exist, and the private health insurance industry would play a significant role. Second, the President reiterated his call for competition as well as regulation as a method for improving the health care system.

In political terms, NHI would provide not only the needed additional benefits but also the political muscle necessary to restructure the health care industry to make it more efficient and more responsive to competitive forces. We think this can be done, and can be made consistent with our present concern for inflation, as long as the program is planned and phased in with the danger of inflation always in mind.

Question Period

Ronald Hurst, Caterpillar Tractor: Could you provide more specifics on cost control under President Carter's NHI plan?

Mr. Onek: We are looking at a wide variety of approaches, ranging from increased regulation to methods for enhancing competition. There is no question that the regulatory approach would include new methods for reimbursing hospitals on a prospective basis. We have not yet determined how that would be organized, but in any case, we will no longer have a system where anything a hospital pays for is automatically reimbursed. How to handle physicians' fees is a much more difficult question, both politically and technically. Obviously, we will be looking at fee schedules, but we have to recognize that what physicians earn is not necessarily crucial. The more telling factor may be the resources that they use from the rest of the health care system.

On the competition side, we're looking at ways to encourage greater use of less expensive delivery methods. We have proposed legislation that would make it easier for Medicare-Medicaid recipients to enroll in HMOs and would give them a greater incentive to do so. For covered employees, we would certainly say that an employer does not have to pay more than the cost of the least expensive federally qualified plan in his community.

Finally, we are going to attempt to strengthen the Health Planning Act through cost containment legislation and through our reimbursement system. A whole variety of methods besides direct regulation can make a difference in effective planning.

Robert Hendrickson, Sherwin-Williams: Could you elaborate on the financing of NHI?

Mr. Onek: The administration will try to finance NHI with as little new tax revenue as possible. It would be impossible to do without any new taxes at all, simply because many people are now uncovered and the only way to cover them is through government expenditures. We estimate that this year some $45 billion is spent in private premiums, mostly through employer plans. We do not intend to transfer these payments to the tax rolls by increasing taxes $45 billion. We do intend to rely as much as possible on the existing employer-employee premium contributions.

Walter Unger, Private Consultant: What provisions will be included in the administration's next proposal for hospital cost containment legislation?

Mr. Onek: That will be determined in large measure by what Congress is likely to pass.

Marion Ein, National Health Policy Forum: Has cost containment ever developed grass roots support?

Mr. Onek: Cost containment has never become wildly popular and it is unlikely to, given the nature of the financing system. However, a recent Harris poll listed rising health care costs as the fourth greatest concern of the American people, behind inflation generally, the federal tax level, and unemployment. It seems we have had some success in alerting the public—and the Congress—to the impact of rising hospital costs. We have a very good chance of securing passage of hospital cost containment legislation next session.

Donald Strange, The Center for Health Studies: What is your view of the Voluntary Effort for cost control?

Mr. Onek: We don't think that, left to itself, the VE will succeed. We are not sure that its proponents think so either, since they have opposed so strongly even those legislative proposals that wouldn't go into effect unless the VE fails. Very strong forces linked to the current reimbursement system make any such effort difficult, but we will certainly be delighted if it does succeed.

I would like to add that in evaluating the success of the VE, we must take into account the fact that several states, including some of the largest states, have mandatory programs that have held down costs.

Also, we can't measure the VE's effects only over a very short period of time, because it is very easy to reduce costs in the short run. The question is whether the effort will work over the long run. Of course, we will be delighted if it does.

Michael Soulier, E. I. DuPont: Are there any plans to provide incentives to convert excess hospital beds to other uses and to restrict the increase in the number of physicians?

Mr. Onek: At least one version of the cost containment bill supported by the administration did contain a conversion provision. We intend to address the potential oversupply of physicians in new health manpower legislation.

Winfield Dunn, Hospital Corporation of America: What steps is the administration taking to reduce the cost of health regulation?

Mr. Onek: Many regulations, such as some portions of the life safety codes, may well be more expensive than they are worth. HEW is now looking at both its existing regulations and all proposed regulations from a cost-benefit point of view to try to reduce the burden.

I would add a footnote on the question of the excess costs of government regulations. That argument would be much stronger if those who make it would segregate that portion of regulation that serves no valid social, physical, or safety function, because the other portion is a valid cost. The implication that every government regulation is by definition negative does not serve much purpose. It would be more useful to define those areas where there is thought to be excess.

COMMENTARY

H. Peter Kneen, Jr., Director, Employee Benefits, IBM Corporation

My major concern with proposals for NHI is that they invariably start with the premise that the country cannot do without it. Regardless of which of the many health care–related problems is being discussed—cost control, access to care, sound physical and mental health, and so on—an NHI proposal is often quickly advanced as the appropriate or even necessary foundation for a national health policy.

This is not to argue that some form of NHI may not, in the end, be entirely appropriate. However, we have two such systems already—Medicare and Medicaid—and their histories do not suggest that more NHI would necessarily mean better health insurance or better national health. To be sure, we need better national health policy, but NHI is, at least to me, still a very open issue. The Carter principles would serve to stimulate a much more meaningful dialogue if they could be viewed and discussed in a context outside of their intended relationship to NHI.

As a first step, let's eliminate those of the ten principles that are only needed because of the intended creation of NHI. Principle 6—no additional federal spending until fiscal 1983, followed by phasing, with each successive step reevaluated based on economic and experience considerations—is clearly not needed if there is no NHI. The concept of phasing is commendable in terms of caution and control; it would help make sure that the program is inherently sound and will not be disruptive to other national interests. However, phasing raises the spectre of a long period of uncertainty as to the nature, extent, and timing of actions. This, given the complex set of interrelationships in the health care delivery and financing systems, may be largely counterproductive.

Principles 7, 8, and 10 relate to NHI financing, the role of the private insurance industry, and consumer representation. To the extent that these principles relate to NHI, they are unnecessary without it. As for their relationship to other health policy issues, the private insurance industry already plays a major role in the system and appears anxious to develop new approaches to improving it, and consumer representation is already assured by existing health planning legislation. Another principle that does not appear to require NHI for its implementation is 3, which assures freedom of choice of physicians, hospitals, and health delivery systems. This flexibility already exists. Finally, principles 4, 5, and 9 relate to efforts for containing rising health care costs. A number of efforts are already under way; others undoubtedly can be developed and tried. It is hard to see why NHI, which would probably result in pressure to further increase costs, is needed to give impetus to cost control efforts.

This leaves us with principles 1 and 2, which are essentially the proposed "basic rights" of all Americans to receive quality health care at a price they can afford. It is difficult to take issue with the intent to place these principles at the head of the list. However, in considering both national priorities and specific programs, the debate should not lose sight of other basic rights, such as enough nutritious food on the table every day, a decent place to live, and an education that is adequate to prepare for a meaningful and productive life. What can we say about our nation's success to date in assuring achievement of these objectives? Does our experience here suggest that sweeping national programs produce the most effective solutions? We must examine carefully whether what is needed are specific solutions to specific deficiencies or a broad program that ultimately affects all segments of the health care system and all consumers as well.

COMMENTARY

Irvine H. Dearnley, Vice-President, Citibank

I would like to put forth some observations on the current health care policy ferment, from the perspective of one individual involved in the development of employee benefit plans and the provision of related technical services. They concern the posture of the private business sector with respect to President Carter's NHI principles, the VE, and the advertising campaign by the health insurance companies.

The Carter NHI guidelines represent such an enormous departure from approaches like the Kennedy-Corman Bill, of which the private sector has been so critical, that they deserve more than the half-hearted support they seem to be receiving. It's no surprise that Senator Kennedy and the unions are less than enthusiastic, but the lukewarm response of the business sector is surprising. Some are saying the lack of legislative action on NHI and cost containment implies that both are ideas whose time has passed— that NHI is not needed. It is more realistic to acknowledge that the major elements of an NHI system are already in place: the major insurance programs, Medicare and Medicaid, HMOs, health planning, manpower programs, and state rate review programs.

The choice is between enacting a national system or closing the gaps in the current system. As long as there are groups in our society who are underinsured or not covered at all (the argument over the precise number is beside the point), the problem can't be swept under the rug. It behooves the private sector, then, to take a more active role in seeing the gaps in our present system are filled on an incremental basis and thus to lessen the risk of something much less palatable.

There's a consensus of substance that the VE lacks credibility. Some of the questions being asked by the skeptical are: Wasn't it a hastily conceived, last-minute initiative to block hospital cost containment legislation rather than a good-faith effort? Does it have any real substance other than jawboning, and if so, what is it? How could it possibly have been implemented so expeditiously as to accomplish the results claimed for it almost before it was under way? We've all agreed there's no quick fix in this business! Unquestionably, we'd all like to see cost containment achieved without further regulation. But the record to date isn't good, and doubts concerning the good faith of the VE don't help the situation. Compelling answers for the detractors are urgently needed.

Again, we need positive programs on containing costs from the private sector. It's not enough to say we're for the free enterprise system and against controls: the health care market can't be left to its own devices because it lacks the normal market influences. We've done innovative things before to impact the market; why not in the medical field? Perhaps we should pay surgeons not to do surgery (a surgeon bank like a soil bank) and hospitals to do away with excess beds. (There's at least one report to the effect that Blue Cross is trying this approach.) Once again, we either make the hard choices with respect to hospital charges and doctors' fees or the government will make them for us. And it isn't likely to get done by jawboning and costly advertising campaigns. I recall hearing Paul Ellwood [of InterStudy] say the medical care business is behaving the way we're paying it to behave, and unless we change the incentives it will go right on doing the same things. Further regulation is one way of changing the incentives, and there seems to be a dearth of alternatives with real substance. This brings me to my third point.

Many of us have been disappointed in the response of the third-party payers (insurance companies, Blue Cross, service organizations) to the challenge of health care cost containment. We can't help feeling that it would be more productive if, rather than spending substantial amounts on advertising, insurers would use their financial resources to provide clients with meaningful data on the claims experience of their benefit plans. It's difficult to avoid interpreting the insurers' action as other than, "If you don't want to seriously address the issue, maybe you can talk it to death." The three areas over which many employers have the greatest measure of cost control in the health care area are plan design, financing method, and claims control. Effective claims control is not possible without reliable data identifying the real problem areas. The information needed is basically the same for all employers, so it is even more surprising that it's so difficult to get. I'd like to suggest that providing such data is the single most effective thing the insurance companies could do.

Department of Health, Education, and Welfare Initiatives in HMO Development and Health Promotion

Howard R. Veit and J. Michael McGinnis, M.D.

Mr. Veit: I am optimistic about the future of HMOs. I sense growing support for the HMO concept among business. I personally believe that the success of the HMO movement is dependent on the involvement, support, and interest of the private sector. In recent months, we've spent considerable energy trying to improve the program. Of course, some problems remain.

The existing health care system is an amalgam of small, noncompetitive, inefficient units of production. Although health care regulation and planning are emerging as very positive forces, they are not going to do the job alone. What we need is competition among alternative delivery systems. We need to let the free market work. I envision a combination of sensible federal regulations that promote competition and the establishment of enough of HMOs around the country to achieve a penetration rate of enrollment of at least 10 percent, if not 15 percent, of the population. This would trigger other competitive factors in the health care system and, I think, would serve to control health care costs at least as well as, if not more effectively than, all the health care regulations that government can impose.

We think that HMOs provide an appealing alternative for both physicians and consumers. Existing evidence indicates that HMO members are satisfied consumers and that disenrollment caused by dissatisfaction with the HMO is very limited. HMOs provide consumers with a better deal in their health care than they are getting now on a fee-for-service basis because the prepayment mechanism acts as an incentive to optimize scarce resources. Total premium and out-of-pocket costs for HMO enrollees are 10–40 percent lower than those for comparable people with conventional health insurance. HMOs also promote cost savings in the fee-for-service sector by increasing competition.

HMOs also benefit providers. Many physicians welcome the end of administrative headaches, the freedom to practice medicine without the distraction of having to run their own businesses, the collegial atmosphere, the opportunity for peer review, and the intellectual stimulation that one gets from working in a group.

Most people involved in the very difficult business of getting an HMO started seem to find the same thing: that enrollment tends to start out very, very low. The HMO concept, frankly, is a hard one to sell initially. However, I think that many HMOs are going to find, as they build momentum and a group of satisfied consumers, that penetration will increase over time.

We think, based on the very positive experience with HMOs, that the federal demonstration project for HMOs is now over. Congress, as you know, recently closed the experimental chapter of our history with a significantly expanded legislative authority. HMOs are now viewed as a voluntary private-sector-initiative—an effort which needs to be equally sponsored vigorously by the public sector.

I would like to run through some of the main features of the recent HMO amendments of 1978. The amendments provide $164 million for HMO development over the next three years, which represents a significant expansion. Also, they increase, as of 1980, the total level of operating deficit loans to HMOs from $2.5 million to $4.5 million. In addition, federal loans can be used to finance construction of ambulatory care facilities—the inability to finance these facilities represented a very significant problem in the past. Finally, we are quite pleased that Congress authorized us to provide funds to organize and implement a major national training program for HMO managers. The most serious problem in the HMO business is in finding experienced, sound, solid managers to run our developing HMOs. We are now in the process of preparing to implement the new authority and we are developing general approaches to management training; we would welcome suggestions from industry.

Another facet of our HMO initiative is a new promotional campaign. We are beginning to increase awareness of the HMO concept and to stimulate interest in developing HMOs at the local level. Also, soon we will be appointing a group called the National Industry Council for HMO Development to coordinate business and labor in promoting HMO development in local communities around the country. We've also aimed at a small number of corporations, trying to interest them in supporting development of an HMO.

Mr. Leo Beebe, a former Ford Motor Company executive, has been serving as our ambassador to the business community. Leo and I have been working with the National Executive Service Corps, a group of retired business executives. We hope to establish a way of mobilizing the considerable talent in this group to help us in developing HMOs.

Obviously, we also direct a significant portion of our promotion effort toward physicians. Working with the American Medical Association, the American Group Practice Association, the National Medical Association, and others we'd like to convince physicians that the HMO concept makes sense for them. Organized medicine traditionally has been opposed to HMOs, but I think the climate is changing.

In our ongoing work with HMOs, we are trying to improve their record of compliance with regulations. We are developing a system whereby the fiscal viability of qualified HMOs will be monitored very frequently. Like practically all small businesses, HMOs usually run into some financial difficulty during their first few years. We have to identify those problems early on and mobilize the resources to provide help. Also, over the next twelve to eighteen months, we will institute a quality assurance program in federally qualified HMOs. This program, which we developed in cooperation with a panel of physicians and state regulators, has two components. The first is a set of standards that HMOs will have to comply with in conducting their own quality assurance programs. The second is an external quality assurance assessment whereby an independent outside group will periodically compare HMOs against standards that the HMOs and the federal government develop together. We do not intend, however, to overregulate the HMO industry. There is a very fine balance indeed in developing the financial and the quality-of-services surveillance systems that we need to provide industry with the assurance that a federally qualified HMO is operating properly, but on the other hand not burying the HMO in paperwork that would interfere with its services.

Many challenges are ahead of us. My office just completed a major market survey of every standard metropolitan statistical area in the country. We plan to target on specific communities to get HMO activity started or strengthen existing HMOs. We will be approaching industry in each of the localities to solicit support. Our goal is to establish nationwide average enrollment in HMOs of at least 10 percent. Once the 10 percent penetration is achieved, competitive forces will begin to appear and to have a very significant impact across the country on the problem of health care costs.

Dr. McGinnis:

The President and the Secretary of HEW decided early in the course of this administration that the best way to decrease costs and to improve health is quite simply to prevent disease and disability. My task at HEW has been to participate in the formulation of policy for disease prevention and health promotion in the broadest sense, with particular emphasis on health promotion.

There are known things we can do to prevent disease and disability. For instance, we have known for quite a while that many of the acute injuries that occur in the workplace and elsewhere are preventable, and we are beginning to learn what can be done to prevent chronic diseases. Our efforts in disease prevention and health promotion heretofore have not been particularly strong, consuming less than 4 percent of our federal health budget. I would like to deal with a few activities that we have undertaken in the past ten to twelve months to strengthen our prevention program.

We began by undertaking the first inventory of HEW prevention activities. We subjected that inventory to a fairly intensive review by our own departmental authorities and by a group of experts assembled by the Institute of Medicine. We took the recommendations that grew out of both those reviews and developed a report that includes a series of budgetary proposals to strengthen HEW's commitment in this area.

This policy effort has been paralleled by a number of program activities. We are now completing what will be the essential components of a national health promotion program. Among these are a national health information clearinghouse, a series of regional forums on health promotion, and a number of major initiatives in the areas of nutrition, smoking, alcoholism, and immunization. We recognize the necessity to develop an integrated approach through targeting certain key settings: the school setting, the community setting, the home setting, the medical treatment setting, and, most important, the work setting. The work setting touches 90 million people daily, and it is a place where our health promotion activities can be much more creative and effective.

We are developing a series of state-of-the-art papers about each of the various kinds of workplace health promotion activities, such as hypertension screening, smoking cessation programs, and alcohol abuse programs. We hope to develop a series of models that will apply to different settings and deal with a number of problems. We have had good cooperation from the business community in this effort, and we anticipate that because of this cooperation it will be a particularly successful one.

Question Period

David McIntire, General Mills: Mr. Veit, my company has had very good experience with our two HMOs in Minneapolis. Over a five-year period, employee participation has gone from 20 percent to 60 percent. We are not pushing the HMO option with our employees, but we try to do a good job in communicating the concept to them. There are other large corporations within the Twin Cities who also have 50 percent or better participation. There are several reasons why this is happening. We have a very concerned and interested business community in the Minneapolis-St. Paul area, several corporate medical directors who are supportive of alternative health care delivery systems, and a number of well-established group practice medical centers who wanted to experiment with the concept.

Frank Finkenberg, George B. Buck, Consulting Actuaries: Business has not always responded appropriately to HMOs. On the one hand, many businesses have an antipathy toward HMOs, and, regardless of the federal laws and regulations, have been successful in avoiding any involvement. On the other hand, we find many businesses taking a position of blind compliance with the HMO Act and regulations. This is harmful to HMOs in several ways. For one thing, these firms with policies merely to comply with the law will tend to avoid nonqualified HMOs and may therefore be avoiding some high quality HMOs. They also miss the opportunity to make the HMO responsive to their own needs, because they won't negotiate with it. Further, these blind compliers take a very substantial risk of being involved with HMOs that will fail. Employers should take a constructively critical attitude toward HMOs—become familiar with them, analyze them, and negotiate with them. Employers have a great responsibility and a great opportunity to help make HMOs better, but they have not done this so far.

Mr. Veit: I agree with your recommendation. One of our problems is HMOs' level of competence in marketing. Many don't make the appropriate sales pitches to business and don't enter into negotiations in a constructive way. We also have some employers who are downright apathetic to the marketing approaches by HMOs—the problem really is on both sides. We need to be much more aggressive in the future about training HMOs to market.

Harry Cain, American Health Planning Association: Are there any efforts under way or planned to educate HSAs concerning HMOs?

Mr. Veit: HSAs are one of the groups we intend to focus on. They represent both an opportunity and a potential roadblock to HMO development. We can promote HMOs to physicians and we can promote them to industry and labor, but if the planning bodies such as health systems agencies are posing obstacles, it will be very difficult.

Kenneth Morrissey, FMC Corporation: Do HMOs have any special exemption from HSAs' right to review all federal grants in their area?

Mr. Veit: All grant applications must go to the HSA for review and comment prior to any funding decision; the HSA thus has input, but not the power to approve or disapprove.

Q.: Perhaps the employer's maximum contribution to an indemnity plan should be its premium or subscriber payment to a local HMO. In the auto industry, this would mean a very substantial employee contribution to remain in an indemnity program. What is your view, Mr. Veit?

Mr. Veit: I know of at least one major company that has done that. HMO savings are substantial and the employer would like to reduce his contribution to the indemnity package so that it matches that of the HMO. I certainly think that is a valid reflection of competition. However, such a scheme would probably not be favored by the federal government because it is often viewed as unfair competition to the indemnity system.

Arthur Lifson, Equitable Life: What is your view of for-profit HMOs? The profit motivation might help solve the problem of attracting competent managers.

Mr. Veit: I support for-profit HMOs, and I would like to see how they compare with the nonprofits.

George Bates, M.D., Owens-Illinois: Our experience in Toledo was that physicians were initially uneasy about HMOs, but they changed their minds after becoming involved. In fact, our major problem has not been physician opposition, but the slowness and complexity of dealing with the federal government.

Mr. Veit: We intend to improve that.

Willis Goldbeck, WBGH: Dr. McGinnis, what is the role of labor in prevention programs at the worksite?

Dr. McGinnis: In this area, there is optimal opportunity for business and labor to work together. We are having a paper developed that reviews labor's special concerns about activities of this sort at the worksite. Health promotion activity could provide very fertile ground for the development of a coalition of labor, management, and government.

Ronald Hurst, Caterpillar Tractor: Will these worksite programs dovetail with OSHA?

Dr. McGinnis: We would like to see the initiative for these efforts come from the business community. The government can help in the information-sharing effort and in bringing together representatives from business and other groups to develop the models most useful to you. We do not want to set up another regulatory agency or mandate activities.

Jane Metzroth, J. C. Penney: Do you have any advice about establishing prevention programs for an employer with close to 3,000 locations?

Dr. McGinnis: We don't have easy answers for that, but we hope that our series of models will be applicable not only to the small enterprise, but also to the large enterprise with multiple sites. And, we anticipate identifying some funds for evaluation of current programs so that we can develop a better understanding. I can't emphasize enough that we aren't going into this with any pat understanding or prescription of what ought to be done. We are hoping to develop approaches in cooperation with the business community.

COMMENTARY

Philip R. Lescohier, Consultant, William M. Mercer, Inc.

The main thrust of Mr. Veit's talk was to urge employers to apply their managerial talents to the organization and promotion of HMOs where needed. A joint effort of government, business, and organized labor, he said, will be required to achieve the goal for the 1980s of having 10–15 percent of the population enrolled in HMOs.

There is a serious question whether the growth in prepaid plans that Mr. Veit envisions will come about through the joint private-government effort described, or through local initiatives by community groups, business, and the medical profession operating outside the HEW program. There is further serious question whether the growth will come in the closed-panel HMOs urged by Mr. Veit or primarily in nonqualified independent practice associations (IPAs).

There are several reasons to believe that during the 1980s,

development of nonqualified IPAs is likely to outpace the development of closed-panel plans both in number of plans and in enrollment, at least in the central and southern regions of the country. A description of what might be considered a prototype nonqualified IPA perhaps best reveals the reasons this is the likely course of events. Such plans have the following characteristics:

1. They provide essentially all the benefits of a qualified plan, typically deleting only the dental benefits for children and the vision examination required in qualified plans. They provide a very limited in-hospital psychiatric benefit, and place heavy reliance on an outpatient psychiatric benefit to deliver adequate, cost-effective psychiatric care. This permits them to avoid the excess costs of qualified plans in the psychiatric area that result from the difficulty of controlling the duration of psychiatric hospitalizations. They also provide an inpatient substance abuse benefit, usually limited to thirty days with a required nonconfinement period of perhaps ninety days and coupled with a comprehensive outpatient substance abuse treatment program. This benefit structure in the substance abuse area has proven itself from the standpoint of effective treatment and cost control.

2. They pay 80–85 percent of doctors' fees on a periodic basis, with the reserve generated by the holdback used to cover the hospital fund deficit, if any, and other contingencies that may arise, such as excess utilization of outpatient diagnostic tests and procedures. Physicians' fees may be prefiled, but payment of usual and customary fees, as established by fee profiles, is common and preferred by most doctors.

3. A risk factor of this magnitude, 15–20 percent, is seen as necessary to provide the IPA with sufficient leverage to control hospital utilization. This risk factor is commonly exercised by requiring advance approval of admission of all nonemergency cases, by monthly financial reports to the doctors, and by peer review of the outpatient practice of those doctors deviating from community norms.

4. By contract, each participating doctor agrees to accept the IPA reimbursement as full reimbursement for services. Thus the doctor's office is relieved of patient billing and the necessity to prepare insurance forms for patients.

5. The IPA contracts with employers on the basis of experience-rated monthly contribution rates, guaranteeing such rates for

twelve months. Rates currently quoted by successful IPAs in the Middle West are 10–15 percent under premiums for high-level indemnity plans.

IPAs have demonstrated the ability to enroll 10–20 percent of the groups to which they are offered on their first enrollment and to quickly achieve 20–35 percent penetration. These plans can be developed and provided with necessary working capital for a nominal amount as compared with closed-panel plans. Consequently, they can be funded prior to implementation out of community resources. Generally, all or most funding is provided by the medical community, local employers, local community groups, or a combination of these sources.

In light of the above characteristics, the appeal of the nonqualified IPA is substantial for each player involved. For doctors, there is greater local control and relative freedom from governmental reporting and regulatory requirements, plus reduced administrative and bad debt cost in their own private practice. For the employer, there is the opportunity to negotiate a benefit package that equates with his indemnity plan but with added extensive outpatient benefits, including preventive health services. If the IPA is properly structured and managed, he may expect lower cost through the experience-rating mechanism than he currently pays for a high-level indemnity plan. Most important, he can expect sufficient enrollment to generate a significant saving in one to three years. For the administrator, there is the freedom to design benefits to meet local competition and to avoid wasteful benefits such as long-term inpatient psychiatric coverage.

For the employee-member, there are several advantages and no disadvantages. Most important, office treatments for the entire family are provided without cost by the family physician of his or her choice. Many employees spend in excess of $100 annually, and some a great deal more, for office visits for their family. The opportunity to obtain these services at no cost from the physician he or she prefers is the unique advantage of the IPA. Another advantage is the greater freedom to change physicians. Finally, there are no claim forms to file.

Everything considered, I believe that a rapid increase in both urban and rural nonqualified IPAs can be expected in the next decade. These will be sponsored by businesses, medical foundations, county medical societies, hospitals, and varied combinations of these groups. Collectively, these efforts will represent, in my judgment, the most significant private sector response to the challenge of increasing the efficiency of quality medical care delivery during the 1980s.

COMMENTARY

Ronald H. Kilgren, Employee Insurance Department, Ford Motor Company

At the outset, I want to underscore and support Mr. Veit's comments about the need for competition in the health care industry and the valuable role that HMOs can play. Increasingly, I have become convinced that competitive forces offer more hope for effective cost control than regulatory approaches. It is encouraging to have some acknowledgment from the federal sector that this may be the case.

Competitive influence can generate the key ingredient that regulatory approaches lack, namely, *self*-motivated providers of care who want to make their system competitive in both cost and quality terms. This, in my opinion, is one of the more compelling reasons for business to support the development of high-quality, cost-effective HMOs. Many business people tend to be pessimistic about the overall cost-containment value of HMOs because of the limited initial penetration of new HMOs. I must admit that membership growth for new programs in areas without prior significant HMO activity is usually very slow. However, with assistance from employers and other community interests in the development and aggressive marketing of quality, cost-effective programs, I believe new plans can achieve steady growth. We should not underestimate the impact that a 5–10 percent enrollment in cost-effective HMOs will have on the cost-competitive behavior of traditional fee-for-service providers.

This ripple effect can be substantial. The introduction of successful, cost-effective HMO operations into a high-cost health care market provides a benchmark that otherwise does not exist, raises the awareness among providers of alternative delivery and organization approaches, provides the stimulation to competitive response, and helps overcome the inertia that otherwise prevails. We are all prone, I suspect, to perpetuate the familiar, tried-and-true, comfortable approaches to any business, whether it be manufacturing, sales, government, or health care delivery. Changed economic behavior comes more readily, I believe, when motivated by competition. Providers have historically competed on quality, delivery capability, and sophistication issues rather than costs. If high-quality providers can be brought to participate in successful HMOs, the result can be the addition of that missing pressure to be concerned with cost and price competition.

All this is more easily said than done, of course. The development of quality, cost-effective HMOs in high-cost areas that do not have significant HMO activity is no easy task. Business can contribute significantly, and I believe the most valuable assistance is not in financial support but rather in management expertise in the development and launch phases. Areas of loaned expertise should include market research, socioeconomic and demographic research, financial planning, facility planning, organizational planning, systems development, and public relations. Fledgling HMOs cannot afford to staff up in these areas, and yet a lack of sound efforts here can result in ill-conceived plans and consequent failure. The time and energy requirement for business participants in such activities can be substantial, so I would not understate the true cost to business.

Mr. Veit commented on the need to attract the physician community to the prepaid practice movement and related HEW's efforts in this area. I concur in the need to address this problem and would suggest that hospital managements be added to the target group. I doubt, however, that such groups will react very positively to overtures from the federal government. This is another area for business and can be the most important and time-consuming aspect of developing a new program. It requires considerable effort toward communication, understanding physician perspectives and problems, and working out mutually acceptable solutions. Physicians and hospitals are more likely, I believe, to respond positively to efforts by local business leadership toward involvement in new HMO ventures than to federal efforts.

Business can also help greatly in financial support issues. Personally, I don't feel a plan should be launched that cannot achieve solvency in a reasonable period and repay loans needed to underwrite launch deficits. Business leaders can assist new plans in obtaining long-term financing from lending institutions. Lenders are more likely to help new HMOs whose development and ongoing success have the active support of established business interests.

The enrollment penetration issue deserves an additional comment. I believe employers, including ourselves, have probably overemphasized open enrollment performance and have not given adequate attention to the highest potential source for new HMO enrollees—new hires. New hires tend to be young people forming new households. They will benefit most from HMO coverage and are the least likely to have established ties with a physician or hospital. Companies with significant hiring volume owing either to growth or turnover should examine their new hire processing procedures to eliminate any obstacles or bias against HMO selection. They may be surprised to find that simple procedural changes coupled with an ability among employment people to handle questions about HMOs in an unbiased manner can produce significant enrollment volume in HMOs. Such volume might, in fact, substantially exceed that achievable in highly promoted annual open enrollment efforts.

Mr. Veit's comments on quality assurance regulations raised some concerns. I must admit that I alarm easily when federal agencies announce the development of new regulations, but the negative effect of existing federal requirements on HMO competitive ability bears out my concern. I want to encourage HEW to work with the HMO industry on this effort to avoid building an additional layer of administrative expense which adds to HMO costs that must be absorbed by consumers. In particular, HEW should make special efforts to avoid duplication and overlap with the states, who have primary responsibility for licensure and quality assurance requirements.

Perhaps there is some pressure on HEW from business interests to develop monitoring capabilities that ensure against HMO failure. That is not practical, in my opinion. Mr. Veit's remarks about expecting some failures as a natural consequence of market forces and the small business nature of HMOs should be heeded by business. Companies can help avoid involvement in failing HMOs through participation in their development, or where that is impractical, through a thorough review prior to offering new programs. I might add that involvement in the development of new HMOs provides an excellent experience base for evaluating their programs.

As a closing observation, I was generally heartened by Mr. Veit's comments because they reflected a more practical orientation of the HMO program in HEW than I believe has been the case and a focus on appropriate objectives. I would encourage continued efforts to work with the private sector. In the long run, I am convinced that significant growth in cost-effective alternative delivery systems will be the result of private sector initiatives with a minimum of federal involvement.

COMMENTARY

H. Peter deLisser, Director, Health Programs, The Executive Health Examiners Group

Dr. McGinnis reported that in HEW's approach to disease prevention and health promotion, mental health was considered one of some fifteen priority problem areas. The list also includes smoking, nutrition, alcohol abuse, and so forth.

Our experience at Executive Health Examiners indicates that companies are already willing to invest in basic health promotion programs. Most companies provide annual diagnostic physicals for many levels of personnel. They expect that people examined by our physicians will discover things about their health and follow the physician's recommendations. In addition, many of our clients are glad to have our nurses run monthly health promotion programs in the on-site medical units we operate for them. But when it comes to discussing programs for emotional health, they often call a halt. Physical health programs are supported and encouraged, but emotional health programs are still in the closet.

Ironically, a majority of the physical ailments presented to our examining physicians during an examination have no apparent organic origin. In our nurse-operated medical departments, about 40 percent of the employee visits per month involve health counseling rather than medical treatment. These experiences suggest emotional health should not be just one of the fifteen areas HEW is reviewing; it should be one of the top priorities.

The image of mental health services as being for "sick" people needs correction. Mental health needs to be reviewed at least annually just like physical health. The 90 percent of people who are mentally well could increase their efficiency and stability by knowing how to better handle their disruptive teenager, by communicating more clearly with a dying parent, by modifying their own behavior in a deteriorating marital relationship.

HEW should promote mental health checkups. Through an educational campaign, it should advise people to consult with a specialist in mental health, not for probing and reviewing past experiences, but to identify current life stresses, explore alternative ways of managing stress, and develop and implement plans for coping with stress. HEW might make better use of their funds by making mental health the number one priority.

Congressional Health Policy: The Years Ahead

Lawrence C. Horowitz, M.D., John J. Salmon, and Stanley B. Jones

4

Dr. Horowitz: One of the more irrational aspects of legislating is that we have a committee called Health and Scientific Research that has jurisdiction over everything to do with health—*except* anything that has to do with financing of health care, Medicare, and Medicaid; anything having to do with the veterans' health system; anything having to do with the Defense Department's health system; anything having to do at all with child health; anything having to do with family planning. However, we do have jurisdiction now, jointly, over health insurance legislation and over cost containment legislation.

One of the major questions facing all of us is to decide what is the appropriate role of the federal government vis-à-vis the private sector. How much regulation should there be? How much deregulation should there be? We're going to be rewriting the drug laws, the food laws, and the cosmetic laws, and we're going to have a serious run at health insurance. Regulations are a heavy component of each of those.

Our thinking has undergone a considerable evolution over the past four years concerning the relationship between the committee and the pharmaceutical industry, and it's an instructive tale. Our subcommittee was guilty of paying too little serious attention to the views of the business community in the initial development of drug legislation. We undertook reform of areas that have major impact, not only on the lives of the American people but on the economic health of the nation, and we did it without a sufficient understanding of the dynamics of the business side or an appreciation of their concerns. The business community in turn paid too little attention to the problems the subcommittee was raising.

Thus we used to have some sort of major confrontational session with the drug industry week after week in the committee hearing room. The turning point in that relationship came when the pharmaceutical industry invited Senator Kennedy to speak to their annual meeting. In the past two years we have worked much more closely with that industry, because in drug regulation the health of the American people is tied in with the health of the private sector. The research capability and the incentive for investment in research holds the key to whether we are going to have a continuing supply of effective drugs in this country. Any change in the regulatory process that makes it more difficult to get a drug on the market, makes it more expensive, or requires more time has enormous consequences, not only for the business of the pharmaceutical industry, but for the health of the people who depend on it. We have differences with the industry, but what we also have with them is a continuing, intensive, effective, dialogue. The model of interaction that we have established there is a positive one, and one that shows our concern about the legitimate needs of the business community. I hope when we move on the national health insurance issue that we can develop the same kind of working relationship.

We have not developed or introduced NHI legislation, but only a tentative outline. It indicates a change in policy that says "There is role for the private sector." We are sincere in asking for your help in structuring that role. Through a very slow and painstaking process, the Coalition on National Health Insurance has changed its position. They now say that they can accomplish what they would like to see done for the American people with a role for the private sector and a minimized impact on the federal budget. Those two changes can be seen by industry as positive, as hopeful, and as deserving of a constructive response. The poles have moved toward the center, and the time for serious discussion is upon us. That doesn't mean that we are going to pass NHI in the next Congress, but it does mean that for the first time we have made a serious effort to put together a coalition that will respect everybody's interests.

We on the Health Subcommittee are looking at a whole series of regulatory issues. We need help in that. We have benefited enormously in the pharmaceutical area from having an understanding of how that industry operates. We need to develop for health issues in general a true working relationship with industry.

Mr. Salmon:

Membership changes and jurisdictional issues in Congress will make it increasingly difficult to enact new legislation next year. The House has a particular problem with leadership changes in the health area, since both the health subcommittees will probably have new chairmen in 1979. However, one continuing issue they will have to face is the administration's effort to enact hospital cost containment legislation.

The insurance industry is probably the only constituency in the world for hospital cost containment. It was largely because of a lack of other support that Congress did not move on the proposed hospital cost containment legislation last year.

I would like to review the history of that, and also define the role of our subcommittee of the Ways and Means Committee in the Voluntary Effort. The Subcommittee on Health spent a rather frustrating summer in 1977 trying to develop hospital cost containment legislation that was satisfactory to the administration and could also muster the necessary majority in the committee. In October the health industry came to our chairman, Congressman Rostenkowski, and said, in essence, "We would like to solve this problem ourselves and keep government off our back." Mr. Rostenkowski replied, "We'd very much like to have you solve this problem yourselves so we wouldn't have to put government on your back." That was blown up into a "challenge" to the private sector. What surprised me was that industry came out with very, very specific goals in a December press conference as to what they hoped to do in 1978 and 1979 and future years with respect to moderating hospital costs.

We were also surprised when we sat down with the HEW actuaries and found that the VE could save in the first year as much money as we would have saved under the administration's proposal. The catch was that Mr. Rostenkowski is a very firm believer that voluntary restraint does not happen without some appropriate stimulus. The incentive that he decided to advocate was a backup control program, where if the rate of increase in costs did not go down by the 2 percent set out in the VE guidelines, then controls would go into effect at the end of the year.

Our subcommittee thought that this was a good compromise, and if we had moved very quickly when it was first proposed, we think that such legislation might have carried quite easily in the House. Unfortunately, the health industry started doing some calculations of their own and realized that they had put themselves in a rather tight box. As one industry spokesperson put it informally, "We have to oppose your compromise more than the original bill, because yours has a chance of passing." As a result, we went through the rest of the year in the House fighting the industry tooth and nail, and in the end there was no legislation.

What will happen with cost containment next year is not clear. While I think the administration is still committed to hospital cost containment, they are going to be hard pressed to move their legislation early in the year. So far, the industry's VE figures are somewhat encouraging. It's troubling to note that we can't pinpoint exactly why hospital costs are going down, but the mere fact that they have gone down for seven or eight months in a row is going to make it very difficult for the administration to come back early in 1979 and argue forcefully for hospital cost containment.

Mr. Jones:

The country is entering a new era in health care policy, and this era will have four characteristics.

At long last we may focus on the problems that exist in the real world, rather than seeing Washington as the problem. Ten years ago we were involved in a series of hearings whose major issue was, Is there a problem in the health care field? We went all over the country and many institutions told us that if Washington will go away, there will be no problems. But at this point, it is clear that we all have a problem, wherever we sit, and the biggest part of that problem is rising costs.

Another characteristic of the new era is acknowledgment that the problems are shared by the public and private sectors. The government's biggest health care problem is rising costs, and that's not unlike the problem that private industry is facing. Rising costs are the source of most of the pressure in this country for health care reform or further government action on health care.

A third characteristic of this era is that there will be no bill passed that purports to solve all these problems, or even no one bill that takes a major crack at them. The politics of our day is for less government intrusion and smaller government budgets. I think the recent proposal for NHI from the unions is an acknowledgment of that current political reality. In fact, we are facing a time where giant proposals to reform health care will no longer be talked about in Washington; the proposals will be much smaller and they will take on pieces of the problem one at a time.

Finally, I suggest that we are moving into an era of negotiation rather than one-sided government action. The change in the political realities and the narrowing of the poles of the debate on NHI will make that negotiation much easier.

Given these characteristics of the new era, I believe that we will see in the next few years a strong *threat* of major legislation from the government. I don't think the health care system can be left unchanged and costs continue to rise at current rates without bringing on a cataclysm. So there will be a threat of legislation, and the possibility of a run at NHI in the Senate and in the House has to be taken very seriously, but I think it will prove to be only a threat—and that there will be a hiatus in major legislative action.

If this sort of hiatus in the big bill approach to the problems goes on for a while, the major social challenge this country will face is to come up with a new set of institutions or institutional relationships that allow for some regulation, some restriction of freedoms that all the institutions involved have cherished, and at the same time leave some latitude for creativity and competition that might, in the long run, pay off by stimulating better approaches to health care. We have an opportunity for public-private negotiation and cooperation that we haven't had in a decade.

From the private sector, I would hope that there will be increased interest in sitting down at the table with institutions that had previously been hard to work with because of their political stance. I would hope that some way of addressing their common interests might be found. Work on health planning is a good case in point.

Question Period

Judith K. Miller, National Health Policy Forum: How flexible are the union supporters of the outline for NHI proposed by Senator Kennedy?

Dr. Horowitz: Unions are only one component of the coalition, of course, albeit a critical component. Any legislation will always require a good deal of give and take in the Congress.

Henry DiPrete, John Hancock: Is the wage-based premium included in the outline cast in concrete? It would eliminate experience rating in health insurance and therefore reduce the incentives for large employers to undertake their own cost containment activities because their own costs would not be affected.

Dr. Horowitz: The principles represent a broad outline of our approach—universality, comprehensiveness, cost controls, quality controls, systems reforms. The principles are firm, but the method of achieving them is not fixed in concrete. You cannot enact legislation like NHI by introducing a bill and expecting that it will remain unchanged to the end. What you fight for is that the product be consistent with the principles you support. We would be delighted to entertain any other effective means to realize those principles. I think it's important to get the wage-based premium out on the table for discussion. It has pluses and minuses, just like any other method.

Ronald Hurst, Caterpillar Tractor: Is NHI in any sense "inevitable," given the "new era" outlined by Mr. Jones?

Mr. Jones: If by NHI we mean one coherent insurance system administered and controlled from Washington, there is a good chance that that never will happen in this country. Many of the other Western industrial countries really have what amounts to four or five or six different things going on, where the government does one chunk of the work, the private sector does another, and there are various things in between. There is still a possibility that there will be one NHI plan, but I think it's more likely that we will end up with a system where there are limits on insurers, requirements placed on employers for coverage of certain kinds, and basic outlines of what that coverage has to include, but where there's a lot of latitude left for different types of insurers, different kinds of provider institutions, and, in fact, some careful intentional room for competition among insurers. The thing that would prevent that, frankly, and cause a more unitary approach to get passed would be for the major institutions that have big stakes in this issue to try to tend their own house and not worry about anything else that is going on in the system. If the insurers manage to worry just about their insurance problems, and the doctors just their problems, and the buyers of care, the unions or employers, just their problems, we probably won't do anything to slow down rising costs. If costs keep rising, there will come a point where drastic steps will be taken the way they were in this country in education and Social Security. WBGH's approach to this is right. I don't think that you should take the pressure off at all, but I would say that the inevitability of a unitary NHI bill has decreased considerably.

Mr. Salmon: There is another dimension, besides less regulation, that leads to this type of cautious look toward the future, and that is the whole financing issue. The Ways and Means Committee next year will probably be redebating Social Security for the second time in two years as new wage base rate and tax rate increases hits. The outcome of that debate has to be linked to a great extent with NHI. No matter how financed, the two are very, very closely related, and the country is showing a great deal of reluctance toward more and more government, more and more Social Security tax, and in fact toward any type of federal financing.

Keith Weikel, American Medical International: Does Congress have a sense of increasing dissatisfaction on the part of the American public with government solutions in health care?

Mr. Salmon: I do not see any increased dissatisfaction. However, I do see increased understanding among members of Congress of health care issues.

Dr. Horowitz: I make a distinction between the government role in general and government regulation. Polls indicate that the American people want the federal government to increase its funding in health care. At the same time, they want regulation held to the minimum level necessary.

Ms. Miller: Can you comment on the tension between many cost containment activities and the antitrust strategy proposed by Mr. Havighurst [chapter 5]?

Mr. Salmon: The magnitude of the cost problem will generate enough political muscle to overwhelm antitrust problems. While there is certainly plenty of room for competitive forces in health care, antitrust as the solution is probably just a passing fad.

Samuel Howard, Hospital Affiliates: I have two questions. First, is there any chance of changing the general cost-based reimbursement system under Medicare and Medicaid?

Mr. Salmon: That could only happen for hospitals in the context of overall hospital cost containment. However, it is possible that some change might be made in physician reimbursement.

Mr. Howard: Second, do you think that legislation to provide a capitation formula for Medicare recipients in HMOs is likely to pass?

Mr. Salmon: I think it could if there were a concerted effort, but there seems to be dissension in the administration as to the desirability of the bill.

COMMENTARY

Judith K. Miller, Panel Moderator, Director, National Health Policy Forum

When Bill Goldbeck asked me to convene a group of people from Congress to talk about the Washington health scene and what's in store for the future, I tried to come up with an appropriate theme. It seemed something like Where to, from here?

Probably the better question would be to ask, How do you get there from here? Listening to what some congressional staffers have to say and others on the program have said, one could easily come away with the impression that you can't get there from here, that the problem of health care costs is just too complex for the government to resolve.

In answer to those concerns, I would like to reiterate something that I have said on previous occasions. If you can't lick them, join them. There is one heck of a lot going on in Washington now. You may not like the proposals or regulations being developed, but you don't have a prayer of changing things unless you're in there fighting. I welcome comments and opportunities such as this to find out how the consumer feels. Most all of us in Washington think there is much greater recognition that the consumer may not be the little gal who sits on a committee somewhere and says, "I belong to this health plan." The consumer, in most people's eyes, is industry. Business is the ultimate payer and the ultimate consumer.

I work in a program that has recently undergone a name change that may have confused some of you. Previously we were called the Health Staff Seminar. We provide in-service education to the key staff people in the Congress and in all government agencies that write or implement health legislation. We now call ourselves the National Health Policy Forum signifying our larger role of bringing people to Washington to talk about local needs, about programs that they are funding, or about how federal guidelines and regulations on legislation affect them. We also have a grant application in the HEW for monitoring health legislative developments in all fifty states. We hope this will give us a much better feel for what is going on out there so that we can foster greater dialogue between state and federal government people. Although I still think of myself as a "Fed" because I once worked in the Senate, I think most of us at the federal level realize more and more that a lot of innovation occurs at the state level. When you hear us talking about the federal scene today, do know that we are also exceedingly concerned about what's going on in the states. As you ask questions, it will be very helpful for us to hear about your experiences at the state and local levels.

My job, as you've heard, is to play broker by bringing people to Washington and taking people from Washington around the country. One of the topics that we often confront is problems created because the legislative scene in Washington is in so much chaos. What are some of the reasons for this? I think that we have a weak executive branch in many regards. The President does not have the best of relationships with Congress. He hasn't learned how to set priorities or to coordinate policies among all the various cabinet members and executive agencies.

At the same time, Congress is in some disarray. Next year in the House of Representatives, fewer than half the members will have been there for more than four years. The problem is that it takes a long time to learn the legislative process and use it well. The large number of new members would not create such problems if it were not for the fact that the leadership doesn't have the same control it once had.

Another factor that has been alluded to is the role of interest groups in health care and, in fact, all areas of legislation. The tenor of the times in Washington is "get in there and fight for what's yours." This means it is interest group against interest group. No one necessarily speaks for the consumer. Since coalitions of interest can be developed around particular issues, the result is that you can't develop a comprehensive policy and expect to get it through very easily.

However, we are developing a much more open legislative process. I also think that we are much more sophisticated about the complexity of issues and how policies developed by one department must relate to the next. Until now we have been dealing with parts of the problem on a piecemeal basis. The concern is, how do you reshape programs to meet existing needs, and how do you define needs five and ten years into the future in order to develop programs at the federal, state, and local level to meet those needs?

COMMENTARY

Kenneth J. Morrissey, Manager, Employee Benefits, FMC Corporation

The panel discussion confirmed my belief that the government's health policy development is terribly fragmented. The executive branch is weak inasmuch as priorities have not been established and the President, after four years, is just beginning to understand his leadership role. The legislative scene is confusing, to say the least. Congress currently has few acknowledged leaders, and future congressional leadership in the health policy area is unknown. It is, therefore, extremely difficult to discern a future direction for policy.

I attach particular importance to the financing aspect of health policy because I believe the government has limited understanding and concern for the business community, which ends up paying over 40 percent of the nation's health bill. Mr. Salmon was most realistic in his view that financing is the most important issue of health policy and that it is becoming a bigger problem each year. As the pie of federal expenditures is divided, other, more important uses of revenue—such as financing Social Security—could have a substantial effect on health policy. Mr. Salmon's impressions surprised and pleased me because of the prevailing attitude that the legislative branch has little concern about the financing of programs.

The business community is very skeptical of any legislative effort toward a concerted governmental health policy because of the government's inability to predict, with any degree of accuracy and credibility, what the actual cost of it will be even next year, let alone five or ten years into the future. Medicare is a prime example. The cost was estimated at $1.5 billion when the program was introduced in 1966; the actual cost for 1966 was $3.5 billion and for 1978, $25.6 billion. Naturally, business becomes very skeptical. This is undoubtedly the reason why business is less than enthusiastic about an NHI plan.

When enacting health care policy for the nation, government very frequently yields to social pressures without fully considering the full cost impact. Government advocates health care cost containment, but at the same time enacts legislation inimical to cost containment. An example is the recent signing of the Pregnancy Disability Amendment to Title VII of the Civil Rights Act, which mandates treatment of pregnancy conditions similar to any other disability. The impact of this has been felt in employee health benefit costs to the tune of billions of dollars. Specifically, the amendment requires unilateral expansion of benefit plans to assure immediate pregnancy coverage upon being hired, regardless of whether conception occurred prior to employment. It also requires short- and long-term disability plans to cover pregnancy situations.

These are examples of how particular health legislation drives up business costs unmercifully. Business people question the cost effectiveness of this and most other health policy legislation. They also question the government's rationale for the allocation of the nation's health care funds. Would it not be preferable to use the monies called for by this pregnancy legislation to provide cata-strophic insurance for the population, or to provide additional funding for HMO development?

I do not wish to imply that social issues are not important—legislators obviously must consider them. Rather, I seriously question whether our legislators realize that health care expenditures must be judiciously allocated on a cost-effective basis. Legislators must become more sensitive to what the nation can realistically afford, keeping in mind that business is the major source of funds for any health policy they might plan. They also must assure that health policy priorities are established and that they are not unduly influenced by specialized interest groups.

Competition or Regulation: The Case for Antitrust Enforcement

Clark C. Havighurst

My current affiliation with the FTC and my general involvement in the antitrust enforcement effort in the health services industry signify a belief that intelligent antitrust enforcement is needed to make that market more responsive to consumers' needs and particularly to their concern—and your concern as employers—about costs. The antitrust approach to the health care cost problem depends mainly on the time-honored prohibition against any collaboration among suppliers that destroys competition. The antitrust laws, as they have developed under section 1 of the Sherman Act, have never, except in the depths of the Depression, allowed competitors to agree to destroy competition, even when the anticompetitive collaboration appeared to have some worthy purpose. This principle was reiterated recently by the Supreme Court in a case involving the engineering profession. That profession had maintained an ethical prohibition against competitive bidding for contracts, allegedly because competition might induce the building of unsafe structures. That case showed that the so-called learned professions can no longer hope to be exempted from the rules of free enterprise, or even to be treated much differently from other business groups.

Antitrust doesn't maintain that competition is always desirable, but it does embody a presumption that the results of a competitive process are preferable to those yielded by private regulation undertaken by an industry cartel. When free competition is not a useful or trustworthy course in a particular market, as sometimes it is not, it is for Congress to declare that fact. In so doing, Congress is in a position to supply a publicly accountable regulatory scheme as a substitute for market forces. Without an explicit statutory exemption, however, private regulation of sensitive matters affecting price and industry output will not be permitted because of the inherent conflict of interests that afflicts those who undertake to regulate themselves. Such private regulation lacks accountability to consumers either through the market or through the political process.

My main purpose in addressing competition and antitrust is to open up discussion of the possibilities for market-oriented solutions to the problems of health policy. Obviously, antitrust cannot by itself solve all these problems, but I think it can make it feasible to adopt a competitive approach in the health care environment. My hope is that antitrust enforcement will soon be able to show some clear success in improving the climate for a wide range of private sector cost containment efforts. And, as that success is increasingly noticed, it may well point the way for adoption of explicitly market-oriented policies—perhaps initially by some HSAs who depart from the usual regulatory approach, perhaps by some state governments, and perhaps even by the federal government.

I don't think that this hope is as unrealistic as it may seem. The cost problem is not going to go away. Government and private interests both will continue to respond to any promising developments that appear. The antitrust enforcement effort really only began in 1975 or 1976 and has involved the effort of fewer than fifty professionals. While I wish we could show more results today than we can from this limited effort, I believe a lot of behavior has been changed and that many things are now possible that were not before. By contrast, the regulatory effort (the certificate of need program, for example) has been around considerably longer and has had much more money and effort invested in it, and I don't think it has shown as many clearly positive results. Meanwhile, the competitive private sector has shown increasing vigor and growing capacity to work constructively on the cost problem. Because Congress is not anxious to take any definitive actions on health care, I think that they would be pleased to see their agenda for interfering with this very difficult and controversial industry shrink a little because the market seems to be doing some of the job.

If you subscribe to the shibboleth that the market doesn't work in health care, you will see my attachment to competition as quaint, and antitrust will probably appear to you as simply a barrier to public-spirited actions, such as the so-called Voluntary Effort, that are proposed to be taken by the private sector. I don't see the matter that way at all. To my mind, real cost containment that gives the public all that it's entitled to can occur only in a market that is not dominated by the medical profession. To embrace the VE, it seems to me, is to confirm and perpetuate the medical profession's power. Such cost relief as one would get under the VE would be only a token, the minimum result that industry interests perceived to be sufficient to prevent the enactment of unwanted regulatory legislation that Congress isn't very anxious to enact in any event.

Surely we should be seeking more fundamental remedies than that. I, for one, wouldn't apologize for using the antitrust laws to challenge the industry's claims that it has the responsibility to solve the cost problem. That claim of authority to regulate is in itself an important barrier to the development of competitive solutions, which alone have the potential to keep providers from continuing to have things their way.

How might the health care sector look under the market alternative? Speculation is necessary because we have never seen such a world and the range of possibilities under this alternative isn't well understood. Government has invested a lot of money and effort in developing, testing, implementing, and evaluating regulation, but comparatively little effort has gone into studying how the private sector might address the cost problem. Moreover, little governmental interest has been shown in health policy measures that would strengthen market forces by doing such things as removing government-created distortions in private incentives, fostering private innovation and useful forms of competition, adjusting such legal constraints as insurance regulation, improving the flow of information, and recasting public financing programs to build on the market's strengths rather than undercutting them.

The one feature of my speculations that distinguishes them from other market advocates' is the greater role I would anticipate for private health insurance and the comparatively lesser role I visualize for HMOs. Such astute observers as Paul Ellwood and Alain Enthoven have offered the HMO as the primary vehicle with which to enforce competition and increase cost consciousness in the health services system. I have gradually lost some of my enthusiasm for that idea, as I have come to recognize that the market has other things to offer.

Moreover, Congress has very nearly strangled the HMO concept by embracing it. Though I still regard HMOs as extremely useful and desirable participants in the marketplace, I find it regrettable that emphasis has diverted attention from private health insurance and its unexploited potential for innovation to meet the cost problem and other current needs.

Almost all the current reform proposals in health care have proceeded on the assumption that private third-party payment is a colossal market failure. Yet private insurers in other fields have satisfactorily addressed similar problems by taking numerous actions to curb the natural propensity of consumers to spend the insurers' money on benefits that aren't worth their cost. Insurance adjusters, multiple estimates, fixed cash benefits, and other mechanisms have been widely used, and it is appropriate to ask why similar mechanisms are so hard to find in medical care insurance. Well, one common explanation is that health care is "different." That is only to say that there are special considerations in this market that make the problem harder to solve, but certainly don't make it impossible.

In my view, the market that should concern us is not insurance, but overinsurance; that is, overbroad coverage, overliberal claims payment policies, and overpermissive attitudes toward providers. Overinsurance is traceable in large measure to the tax laws' treatment of health insurance as a nontaxable fringe benefit, for both income tax and payroll tax purposes. As individuals have become substantially overinsured, the distortions in the demand for medical care that insurance necessarily introduces have been exacerbated.

Without the perversities introduced by tax incentives, health insurance would look very different. Comprehensiveness in benefit packages would not be the ideal it has become. Consumers would have more reason to limit their payments into a premium fund on which others could draw. Heavier coinsurance, larger deductibles, exclusion of both highly discretionary items and minor budgetable items, such as prescription drugs and dental care, would be standard. Insurer efforts to police spending would be much more common than they are today, and would be generally approved. I believe that changing the tax law would be an important step toward new ways of obtaining protection against medical costs.

In addition, private health insurers and others have faced overwhelming resistance from the medical profession whenever they have attempted to take cost control measures. The ever present threat of professional retaliation may well provide an entirely sufficient explanation for the reticence of health insurers in the past to serve their customers' interests in cost containment. But it is becoming increasingly clear that the antitrust laws now prohibit most of the concerted professional activities that have stood in the way of third-party innovations in the past. If those laws can be effective against professional conspiracies, then insurers or others will be free to adopt more aggressive policies toward providers and to experiment in an unrestrained competitive environment with new approaches toward this problem. Antitrust can put the ball in the private sector's court.

The antitrust laws also have a function, I think, in making it clear that consumers and insurance purchasers must look for cost relief primarily to private financing mechanisms, and cannot depend on provider cartels such as the VE. My own sense is that the antitrust laws should stop provider groups not only from directly interfering with private attempts at innovation, but also from organizing their own half-way measures to forestall the growth of new financing and delivery mechanisms.

I recognize the complexity of private cost containment, including not only the difficulty in deciding just what to do, but also the problems in dealing with the unions and the expectations of employees, who take for granted such insurance plan features as comprehensiveness of benefits, free choice of physician, and automatic payment of claims. Industry must find ways of giving employees new opportunities for increasing their take-home pay by taking a different set of health benefits. Gradually, out of the numerous experiments and initiatives that industry undertakes, there should emerge a variety of effective, individually tailored solutions which, in the aggregate, will amount to a major reorganization and restructuring of the health care financing and delivery system.

I would like to suggest one approach out of the many available: the use by insurers of participation agreements with selected individual providers. These contracts should incorporate fee schedules and provisions that would secure physicians' cooperation with the administrative requirements needed to control costs. For example, doctors could be contractually required as a condition of getting paid to submit certain cases for a second opinion, for predetermination of benefits, or for prior authorization by the insurer. A more modest but still extremely promising model is the "health care alliance," a group of hospitals and doctors whose patients pay premiums based on the providers' efficiency. An insurer could easily offer a group of efficient providers the chance to market their efficiency in this way.

I believe that there is much yet to be learned and done about organizing the health sector to achieve cost containment. Our effort must be to encourage innovation by all the private actors—insurers, HMOs, employers, unions, provider groups, and so on—by changing the market environment so that consumer-dictated change, privately initiated, can more readily occur. Government hasn't yet found, and seems unlikely to find anytime soon, an answer to the cost problem that would be widely accepted, and, while it flounders, the marketplace continues to operate. If the antitrust effort is at all successful in facilitating these developments, we may find someday that the private health care system runs well enough that it can be left pretty much alone.

Question Period

Larry Lewin, Lewin and Associates: How can we get around the fact that most large employers pay all or nearly all the health insurance premiums for their employees, short of changing the tax laws?

Professor Havighurst: There are different ways of trying to deal with that. One is to suggest the possibility of changing the policy of paying 100 percent of each employee's benefits. I also like the model of offering the employees first of all a big package, and then offering them the chance to choose something more limited within that and giving them the difference in cash. I think that employers have some obligation to screen the available choices so that they are reasonable choices, but not to put themselves in the place of choosing for the employees in all respects.

Bruce Sidebotham, General Tire and Rubber: Is there still much room left for innovation, given some of the government-mandated benefits and coverages in health insurance?

Prof. Havighurst: I agree that some options have been foreclosed. One just has to function within the legal framework and do whatever is left over. Certainly the HMO Act is the classic instance of a legislature trying to write in all the details they could think of. We've seldom had a clearer demonstration of how Congress just can't make decisions for people. One hopes that when a few things begin to happen, then maybe people can go back to legislatures in the states and get more of these decisions put back into the private sector where most of them belong.

Q.: Isn't union opposition a roadblock to these proposals?

Prof. Havighurst: Every situation will be a little different, and perhaps some things are possible in one setting and not in another. We are paying through taxes or through noncollection of taxes a significant share of a very expensive health benefit package that the unions have somehow decided is a desirable thing. It's quite clear to me that what they are buying for their members is not entirely in the members' best interests, and I would prefer to see the tax law changed so that they would, in fact, bear the full cost. Union leaders seen to feel that health benefits are something that is easy to sell and that enhances their position with the rank and file. I recognize that this is a severe problem, but I also think that some unions would not oppose the offering of competitive alternatives to the rank and file, allowing them to economize in some though probably not all possible ways.

COMMENTARY

Frank E. Finkenberg, Benefit Consultant, George B. Buck Consulting Actuaries, Inc.

Professor Havighurst's message is basically a cheerful one for business: the market system can work for health care, and its failures can be blamed on other things—distorted incentives owing to tax deductibility of medical costs and organized resistance by provider groups to system reform. Further, solutions are to be sought not through regulation or voluntary provider efforts, but in the private sector, through the operation of the market. And who shall lead the way but the much-maligned health insurers.

A response to this message requires a brief look at what the market in health care is like and how it got that way. Is health care "different"? That is, is it immune to market pressures, making nonmarket solutions necessary? With 70 percent of medical costs paid by third parties and decisions as to price and quantity largely made by physicians without the need to consider the patient's ability to pay, one is tempted to agree. The Committee for National Health Insurance certainly seems to take that stand, demanding effective nationalization of health care delivery and financing, while other fundamental human needs can be met through the private sector.

But let's take another look. When the art of medicine was simpler and most care was paid for by the patient, the physician had the primary voice in decisions as to the price, quantity, and nature of services rendered, but his recommendations were tempered by how much the patient could reasonably pay. Charity care was given, but there was still the economic constraint of how much free care could be sustained by contributors and paying patients. The system worked tolerably well. Those days are gone, but one can't point to tax disincentives and provider cartels as the prime villains. The growth in demand for medical insurance, through both the public and private sectors, has been a perfectly rational response to economic and technological developments. The increasing complexity of medical care meant that patients became less competent to participate in decisions as to the necessity, quality, and price of care at the same time as the economic consequences of those decisions became much more important. The monetary stakes were also raised by a change in the most prevalent diseases from acute infectious ones to more costly chronic problems. Health workers also successfully demanded a larger share of national income. The rational response of consumers was to seek protection through insurance from the financial results of costly medical decisions that were beyond their control. They did this by exercising economic power, in demanding employer-sponsored medical benefits, and in the use of political power to bring about Medicare, Medicaid, and favorable tax provisions.

As a result, patients are no longer purchasers of health care. But this in itself did not cause a "market failure." As Professor Havighurst points out, other third-party payment systems work reasonably well, even, I would add, when full insurance is encouraged, as in homeowners and automobile coverage. What set the stage for disequilibrium in health care was that the new purchasers—employers, government, and insurers—have been slow to adopt the informed consumer role, leaving all decisions to be made by providers. Ironically, the one group that most clearly recognizes the link between the obligation to pay and the right to participate in decisions as to the need for treatment and the reasonableness of charges are the supporters of a nationalized system. They would centralize purchasing power in the federal government, and with it the power to determine provider incomes and allocate care.

If a private sector market in health care is to function, the needed innovations will come through employers' actively assuming the role of health care purchasers. I'd put my money on employers rather than insurers for a number of reasons. Most importantly, the insurer doesn't ultimately foot the health care bill; the employer does. Therefore he has the greater incentive to control this rapidly rising expense. Also, the employer is in a strong position to influence patient attitudes, since the patient looks to the employer as the source of all employee benefits, including the most important one, the paycheck.

In the last few years there has developed a thriving market in one segment of health care financing—the administration of employer plans. New financing mechanisms have been developed and new entities and computer systems have arisen to pay claims, all in competition with the traditional approach of insurers. These innovations were developed in response to *employers'* desires to reduce health care insurance costs; insurers were hauled into the marketplace over a barrel.

As evidence of insurers' lack of acceptance of the role of health care purchaser, I would cite their continued emphasis on coinsurance as a cost containment approach. While these provisions have some value, they are essentially an attempt to transfer back to the patient decisions as to necessity, price, and quality that he or she is no longer capable of making and has shown by economic and political votes a strong desire to avoid. One has to wonder why economic decisions made by individual patients who bear only 20 percent of the cost would result in lower health care spending than those made by sophisticated insurers bearing 100 percent of the cost.

From the insurers' point of view, it's a sound business decision not to innovate in health care. One of the scarcest resources in any organization is creative, innovative thinking. Insurers will naturally devote these resources to projects with the greatest ratio of reward to risk. In any ranking of potential projects by this ratio, health care innovation is likely to be near the bottom. In explaining such interest in health systems as they do have, insurers are likely to cite pressure from major employer accounts, fear of increased government intrusion, or a vague concept of social responsibility.

Some employers, meanwhile, have started to get involved in health care for the best of all free market reasons—to maximize profit by containing a key cost of doing business. They have founded or supported efficient, high-quality HMOs. They have audited the claims-paying operations of their insurers or administrators to be sure that their money is well spent. They have demanded meaningful health care statistics—and used them to improve benefit design and to deal directly with providers to reduce costs. And they have made available some health services through direct contracts with providers.

As more employers take these actions and develop new approaches to assert their rights as the true purchasers of health care, the prospect for a private sector market in health care will brighten.

The States and Health Care Costs

Jonathan E. Fielding, M.D.

I would like to report on what one state has done and is trying to do about health care cost inflation and also give you a magic list of ten practical measures that industry can take toward that goal.

It is clear that our current health care system lacks incentives to control costs. Not only are hospitals automatically reimbursed by third parties practically without question, but several studies suggest that the more physicians there are in any area, the higher their fees. So much for supply and demand. The result is that we now spend 9 percent of our GNP on health care, and for many corporations health care premiums are the largest single expenditure. But we're not seeing returns to scale in terms of health status or decreased mortality, and that's where we come in as a state. Everybody's looking to the states, in part, because the federal government has not been effective and because the states are seen as more responsive to local needs.

The states have a strong interest, apart from issues of public good, in trying to control health care costs. Last year our Medicaid costs in Massachusetts went up $100 million with no increase in benefits. Also, many states, Massachusetts among them, are either the largest or one of the largest employers and pay most of the premium costs for their employees. When those go up, the taxpayers must bear the burden, and everybody knows how much our citizenry likes increased taxes.

We've done a few things about this problem in Massachusetts. One is hospital rate setting. Like several other states, we have a commission with the authority to approve prospective hospital budgets. This effort has led to a reduction in the growth of hospital cost in Massachusetts, from 14.6 percent in fiscal year 1976 to 9.3 percent in fiscal year 1979, compared with 15–16 percent nationwide. The other states that have done the same have had roughly the same experience. The slowing of hospital inflation may be more due to state rate-setting programs than to any voluntary restraint. Rate setting, I might add, is not an expensive program. It costs the state only $2–3 million to administer it, though it's hard to determine what it's costing the institutions. However, whatever that actual cost is, it has to be seen in terms of the $2.3–$2.5 *billion* of hospital costs in Massachusetts.

The second thing Massachusetts has is a strong certificate of need program, as required under the Health Planning Act, that reviews all capital expenditures over $150,000 that health care institutions want to make. The Public Health Council, the nine-member decision-making body is tough, but I think fair, and has tried to develop quantitative standards against which to measure applications. For example, they use 3.4 beds per 1,000 population as the standard against which to judge applications for acute care beds. If you look at the lifetime cost discounted at a reasonable rate and brought back to 1976 dollars, the program has saved approximately $2.9 billion over its first five years, and total beds in Massachusetts in the last few years have gone down rather than up.

Massachusetts also has strong health planning, with very good support statewide from all the groups involved. We've looked at managing the growth of nursing homes, because nursing homes are the fastest growing segment of health care costs in Massachusetts. We have also been encouraging outpatient care when it is clearly substitutable for inpatient care. Also, every hospital has to submit plans specifying not only future capital projects but also their impact on operating costs. We look very hard at both costs.

Also in our planning process, we work with the HSAs to get agreement on standards in order to minimize the problems that occur when an HSA says yes or no and the state says the reverse. It's hard, because there's a natural tension between regional agencies that want things for their region and a statewide agency that aims for equity among the regions, but often those points can be ironed out.

The fourth thing we've done is encourage HMOs. We have a state law that facilitates their growth, but also has strict licensing provisions. We are currently spending $200,000 a year to help HMOs get started. We are supporting all types and all sponsorships; in many cases, industry, Blue Cross, or private insurers are involved.

We have also introduced a mandatory second opinion program for Medicaid recipients for the most commonly abused procedures. We can see quality benefits as well as cost benefits as a result.

Finally, we now have a generic drug law that says every physician has to use a prescription form with two signature lines. One says dispense as written; the other says you can substitute a lower priced product. We are encouraging substitutions by talking to industry and consumers and saying, "Ask your doctor why not." We feel that this is going to save millions of dollars in the first year of operation.

I can make a strong case for what we're doing, but it's important to realize that government is fragile. Nobody recognizes this better than I since the incumbent governor was not renominated, and it's unclear what attitude the new governor will have toward these efforts. So it is essential that industry become involved and provide that link of continuity.

Let me set out ten concrete steps for industry:

1. Support strong state regulatory and planning efforts. Make sure that, if your state legislature and governor are generally probusiness, that they are also probusiness on health care issues. This means strong certificate of need, prospective rate setting, and planning standards.

2. Reconsider industry's lack of support for hospital cost controls. There is no market system and little competition in health care, and so you can't assume that the solution to health care inflation is the same as for inflation in the rest of the economy. By supporting cost containment legislation now, industry can carve itself a much greater role in deciding the content of the laws and regulations.

Related to that, the eleventh of my ten points is to encourage limitations on physician manpower. No matter what we do to control inflation, if we have too many doctors, each of whom orders services that account for $250,000 or $300,000 a year, we will have inflation. We are producing physicians at an increasing rate and clearly in excess of need.

3. Be active on the boards of Blue Cross and Blue Shield, the HSAs, and hospitals in areas where you have significant numbers of employees. Industry representatives need to be trained on the issues and shown how they can directly help or hurt their company through their actions.

4. Support the growth of well-managed HMOs. A good HMO should have strong internal controls on utilization and costs and, in general, should have lower premiums than Blue Cross–Blue Shield. I would suggest that you encourage the formation of several HMOs in most areas to get competition into the prepaid health care market and actively encourage your employees to join.

5. Periodically reevaluate your health benefits and consider some of the longer term impacts and trade-offs. In every bargaining cycle there should be an opportunity to increase some benefits and look at others where diminution may be in everybody's interest.

6. Evaluate your system for reviewing and controlling claims. There is still a fair amount of overcharging, questionable procedures, and bad utilization, and most companies and insurers don't have the systems in place to really control these. There are many millions of dollars to be saved in this area. It does mean that some employees won't be entirely happy, but it is in their long-term interest also. We are not trying to save money at the expense of quality—we are trying to have an impact on both.

7. Reduce the frequency of covered or encouraged physicals. The only rationale for yearly physical exams is a particular occupational exposure; the well population doesn't need them so often. Adopt the lifetime health monitoring approach with a minimal list of preventive services provided at intervals according to age.*

8. Install proven preventive medicine programs where the cost-benefit ratio is favorable, even if the effects require several years to show. With experience rating it obviously makes sense to invest in these programs, and besides, well-designed programs may reduce absenteeism and increase productivity in addition to effects on health and health care costs.

9. Whenever feasible, invest in in-house health care programs with salaried or contract physicians. Such a program makes it easier to put preventive medicine programs in place, reduces absenteeism for physician appointments, gives you better control over a disability or a need for hospitalization, and provides a service for employees who don't have to go hither and yon to a number of physicians.

10. Finally, be innovative. There are few clear-cut answers, and I think industry can and should encourage experimentation. What about sharing some of the cost savings resulting from preventive medicine programs with employees? Or putting in incentives such as paying people not to smoke or to control high blood pressure? Industry can try many such approaches and then determine what the impact is.

---

*Breslow, Lester, and Anne R. Somers: "The Lifetime Health Monitoring Program," New England Journal of Medicine 296:601-608 (1977).

Question Period

Q.: What do you think federal cost containment legislation should look like?

Dr. Fielding: The states should bear the brunt of the administrative responsibility. But they should be monitored and if they can't do it, then have somebody else take it over. Also, I think that wage passthroughs don't make sense at a time when workers are being paid in hospitals what they are being paid outside in comparable jobs. If they are not, then perhaps an argument can be made for passthroughs until parity is reached.

Q.: How would you convince management that there is a need to control the supply of physicians, considering management's general belief in the workings of a free market?

Dr. Fielding: It would be harder to argue that market forces are operating today. We have very diverse densities of physicians per 1,000 population in different parts of the country, and even the densest concentration doesn't seem to have influenced prices appropriately. A lot of circumstantial evidence suggests that the prudent policy is not to further increase the physician-to-population ratio.

Peter deLisser, Executive Health Examiners: Perhaps the real value of the annual physical is the health education potential, as opposed to finding specific disease problems.

Dr. Fielding: Health education should be one of the important parts of the physical. The question is if you do a health hazard appraisal and show somebody what their risk is and they don't do anything about it today, what are the chances of their doing it if you remind them every year as opposed to every five years? Also, while I would like to agree with you on the medical benefits of health education, most of that impact has not been well-documented in controlled tests. I am a proponent and a supporter of health education, as you are, but I can't see that changing the frequency of the exam is going to decrease its benefit substantially.

COMMENTARY

John R. Virts, Corporate Staff Economist, Eli Lilly and Company

Regulation, political budgeting, and government control seem so attractive because of the neatness of the apparent resolution of goals and actions—especially when compared with the untidy scrambling of millions of individuals, families, and other groupings seeking to improve their own conditions and pursue their own goals. Rules we need, but every rule affects the result; and, in the end, the results are a consequence of the rules. Health care—costs, access, results—has been heavily influenced by rules imposed and enforced by government: Hill-Burton, Medicare, Medicaid, tax provisions, licensing, manpower training, and so on. The goals sought by every new program and every provision have been based on real concerns for individuals and society. But every program and every provision has also had an impact on the cost of care, the way that cost is borne, and the nature of the care available to each individual.

There seems to be virtually no disagreement, today, with the contention that we need significant changes in the regulation of health care and in the forms of government involvement. Dr. Fielding expresses the belief that state governments and businesses need to accept stronger roles in regulating or controlling health care spending and in developing, promoting, and implementing alternatives, including prevention, to reduce treatment. While disagreeing with many—perhaps most—of his specific prescriptions, I agree completely that the situation calls for action from the states and the private sector.

The sources of recent health care cost increases and the patterns of consumption of health care reveal some of the consequences of inappropriate regulation or control. From 1965 to 1975, total U.S. health care cost increases can be attributed to the following causes:

	Percentage
General inflation, population changes, and new administrative costs	57
Increased real per capita consumption of health care	40
Price increases (primarily following introduction of Medicare-Medicaid)	3
	100

Based on 1970 data, our nation's health care costs are heavily influenced by our caring intensively for a relatively small part of the population—50 percent of the consumption being accounted for by 10 percent of the population. Whatever the forms of regulation and whoever are the regulators, regulation is a form of rationing and must inevitably impact most heavily on relatively few individuals, like those currently consuming great amounts of care.

Today's institutional structure surrounding health care contains, in some circumstances, perverse incentives for providers to drive up costs, as Dr. Fielding and other analysts have noted.

Likewise, many families seek care more readily and monitor its cost effectiveness less stringently than they would under other financial arrangements. However, the existence of such costs— while indicating the need for concern, analysis, and the study of options—does not necessarily signal a need for government regulation at the federal or state level. An absolute minimum first step—one that has not yet really been taken—is sufficient investigation of the magnitude of such costs in order to compare them with the costs generated by changing the regulatory or institutional structure.

Even a recitation by so knowledgeable a regulator as Dr. Fielding of the apparent short-term savings achieved in Massachusetts through reactive and rigid regulation falls far short of the mark of justifying such regulation. For example, a recent study done for HEW* demonstrates that another state (Indiana) has achieved significant cost savings *without* state health department regulation of rates or certificates of need. This is being done with a Blue Cross–Hospital Association–centered prospective rate-setting system designed primarily to operate on the development and utilization of professional management incentives. Such a system is far less likely to generate the long-run costs that inevitably occur under the rigidity of government regulation, even if the regulation occurs on the state rather than federal level.

That perverse incentives for regulators and other forces inherent in rigid, reactive regulation will generate hidden costs is absolutely certain, and the probability is that such costs will be high. Frequently, some of the costs are hidden for years because they are felt only after time passes. One of the effects of the lack of management flexibility, for example, could be a serious inhibition to innovation—and the cost of lost innovation opportunity might never become apparent. Consequently, the forms of regulation proposed by Dr. Fielding need to be tested not only against the criterion of short-run cost effectiveness relative to alternative strategies but also against long-run criteria. A principal difficulty with government regulation at either the state or federal level is that in the political process, the long-run effects on consumer welfare are rarely addressed because of the lack of an effective political constituency.

A specific example of the possible conflict of consumer's short- and long-term interests can be seen in Dr. Fielding's recommendation to states and businesses to pass laws or incorporate

---

* Patrick O'Donoghue, *Controlling Hospital Costs: The Revealing Case of Indiana* (Denver: Policy Center, Inc., 1978).

insurance provisions leading to the substitution of so-called generic drugs for the drugs of the R&D-intensive manufacturers. It is clear that in some cases drugs are available that are cheaper than some that are currently being prescribed and dispensed. It is also clear that cheaper drugs are lower quality drugs, at least sometimes. It is not always clear whether the more costly drugs are superior enough in quality to justify their higher prices—although markets as competitive as those for prescription drugs should be able to make such decisions. It is totally clear, however, that an arbitrary regulatory-type decision directing spending toward the products of one type of firm and away from another type *will* have some effect. In the case of generic substitution, the direction of spending will be toward firms with lesser or no R&D activity and away from firms with higher, or even much higher, commitment to R&D. The effect will be a reduction of R&D spending. The subsequent effects of this reduction—unachieved innovations in cost-effective drug therapy—might never be recognized, especially as a consequence of the initiating action.

Whatever institution it is that designs and implements regulation—federal government, state government, or private sector institution—must find a way to select alternatives after consideration of both short- and long-term costs. Typically with regulation of health care and its costs, the difficult balance will be today's budgets and tomorrow's improvements. Government regulation at the state level, as suggested by Dr. Fielding, is inherently superior to federal regulation for two reasons. First, state governments have better access to knowledge of, and more sensitivity to, actual local conditions. Being closer to the regulated, state government regulation can be, and is more likely to be, more flexible than federal regulation. Second, a total system, however regulated, will be permitted greater diversity under fifty regulators than under one. Therefore, the chances of exposing both better and worse forms of regulation are improved. From some perspectives, state regulation is more costly than federal, but the benefits just mentioned seem, on balance, to be valuable enough to support the prediction that, if government regulation is required, state regulation will provide superior cost effectiveness.

A primary goal of business, labor, consumers, and providers of health care should be to take those steps that can be taken to correct or reduce the forces that Dr. Fielding believes can be handled only by regulation. Effective statewide prospective rate setting can be, and has been, implemented without legislation and certainly can be implemented in a goal-achieving mode rather than in the typical "how to" regulation mode. Management-by-exception utilization review can be, and has been, implemented by risk-holders in public and private programs with professional review against local standards. It is even possible that a combination of education, incentives, and the provision of benefit options might return some of the financial constraints to patients, and thus to providers, for parts of the employed population whose access to care is not inhibited by deductibles and copayments. HSAs, especially if subject to significant community management, including business, can quite probably achieve positive results without relying on the typically rigid certificate of need regulation.

The federal government's budgetary problems resulting from Medicare and Medicaid are, of course, very real. Our current systems of health care financing have led to some economic inefficiencies, especially with the compounding of some of the problems with government intervention and regulation. However, these facts are totally insufficient justification for any further centralization of a system inherently based on personal needs and criteria—simply the lack of important returns to scale in health care delivery should lead us away from federalization or reliance on federal criteria. Dr. Fielding's basic assessment, then, is in tune with the times: we must begin with actions in the private sector and/or at the state level of government, if for no other reason than to gain the time needed to demonstrate the lack of need for federal control of health care to achieve federal budget control of Medicare and Medicaid. On the other hand, many of Dr. Fielding's specific suggestions are the same sort of rigid, reactive regulation being proposed at the federal level. Application of such kinds of regulation by fifty states will be somewhat less oppressive and will provide some greater chance of exposure of their inefficiencies, but why choose the lesser of two governmental evils when the private sector *can* do the job—if it will? The very existence of the WBGH and its programs is evidence that such efforts are under way. Tomorrow's patient should be fervently praying that all such efforts are successful, because the stakes are clearly the effectiveness and cost of his or her care.

COMMENTARY

Henry A. DiPrete, Second Vice President, John Hancock Mutual Life Insurance Company

Most of what Dr. Fielding has recommended can be supported by the insurance industry. Specifically, I applaud his encouragement of:

1. Health planning efforts, including a strong certificate of need program, community involvement, and planning standards.

2. Support for hospital cost containment activities, both voluntary efforts and state prospective rate and budget review.

3. Encouraging the growth of well-managed HMOs, including both closed-panel models and individual practice associations.

4. Cooperation by insurers in the efforts of large employers to re-evaluate and possibly restructure benefits packages to include proven cost-saving features. As Dr. Fielding recognizes, this requires a corresponding employer responsibility to take initiatives to control claims and implement rigorous claims review procedures.

5. The further study and encouragement of preventive health programs and in-house health care programs.

6. Most important is Dr. Fielding's emphasis on the need for innovation in the private sector. This requires freedom from the fear of professional reprisals or governmental strictures such as antitrust enforcement. Innovation and cooperation among all parties concerned and affected by changes in the health delivery and financing system is mandatory if any real improvements are to be effected. Dr. Fielding's reference to such examples as second opinion programs and, indeed, mandatory second opinion programs, the sharing of cost savings with employees as an incentive for cost-conscious decisions, and other incentives for reform are all to be lauded.

I can only criticize what Dr. Fielding did not say. That may not sound fair, but let me elaborate. Problem areas do exist in the regulatory approaches mentioned in spite of Dr. Fielding's glowing reports. Some of these problem areas are:

1. *Certificate of need.* In the past, the Massachusetts certificate of need program has been plagued by what many refer to as unnecessary bureaucratic delays in consideration and approval and a lack of clarity in the procedural and substantive regulations implementing the program. Although there is presently some hope that these problems are being solved, I refer to their existence as an example of how the system can break down and become counterproductive.

Another area where breakdowns in the system can be seen is in specific legislative circumvention of the certificate of need process, such as we have seen all too frequently in Massachusetts. Institutions that were denied a certificate of need under the existing procedures have persuaded the state legislature to pass special legislation exempting them by name from the state certificate of need legislation. To the extent that such efforts succeeded, the whole concept of rationalizing the state health planning process becomes unsuccessful. We should all look to Dr. Fielding and other experts in the area for advice and guidance on how best to confront this problem, which is really an attack on the certificate of need process.

2. *Medicaid program.* Dr. Fielding did not mention the states' massive cutbacks in the levels of reimbursement to providers through the Medicaid program. Although such actions might have superficially laudatory effects on the state on-line budget figures, the reality of the situation is that cutbacks are simply being passed on or shifted to the other types of payers—for indeed, someone must foot the bill. And, as you might imagine, the one left standing when the other players are seated is consistently the charge payer. I recognize that this is a very complex issue and do not mean to imply that Dr. Fielding should be held responsible for its entire solution. I raise it, however, as a logical addendum to his remarks.

The state, as a concerned party, a large employer, and a payer of a significant portion of health care costs, has a responsibility just like the rest of us to face the problems head on and work with us in attempting to find long-term solutions. The state can't simply continue indefinitely to pass along the increased costs of medical care to other payers, along with the problems that are lying at the root of that inflation. Many observers of American health care have come to the conclusion that traditional market forces are either nonexistent or seriously minimized in that industry. Various solutions have been suggested, including altering the system and freeing up some of the present structures so that increased competition and realigned incentives can combine to instill the market forces now lacking. Another approach, which I consider a bit extreme, involves either sole or a substantial level of reliance upon regulatory measures to achieve the same ends. This approach, the logical extension of which is the public utility concept, would, by definition, eventually achieve total control over the health care system and its problems. It does not necessarily follow, however, that the solutions to those problems provided by such a strategy are the most desirable for the consumers and providers of health care.

I am one of the first to admit that a number of the problems in our system are most appropriately addressed through legislative and regulatory means. Hospital cost containment, health planning, and HMO encouragement and regulation are examples of areas where we and other major health insurers have supported partial regulatory approaches. However, too much is not a good thing, primarily because of the dampening effects on innovation and cooperation in the private sector. Competition, on the other hand, if introduced into health care delivery, could go a long way toward providing the needed incentives for cost-conscious decisions, efficiencies, and increased productivity. But let us not be tricked by anyone into believing that either extreme is desirable. The greatest hope for solution of some of the problems noted by Dr. Fielding and others lies in a cooperative effort between the public and private sectors that maximizes the advantages of both while at the same time achieving a proper balance of interests.

The health insurance industry stands ready and willing to continue its participation in this dialogue and a joint effort to reach these goals. We can be both proud and optimistic about the progress that has been made by the private sector and by government intervention. It is in this spirit of mutual experience—rather than mutual exclusion—that I believe further progress can be made.

Private Sector Perspectives

III

Private Sector Cost Containment Initiatives

*Paul M. Ellwood, Jr., M.D., Jan Peter Ozga,
Kenneth W. White, and Paul W. Earle*

7

Dr. Ellwood: There have been some dramatic changes in the attitude of business toward the health care industry in recent years. First, the concern about health benefit policies and escalating health care costs has been moving steadily up the corporate hierarchy. It is not at all unusual now to visit corporations to talk about health care and to be met by the chairman or the chief executive officer who exhibits a remarkable sophistication about the health care issues facing his company and community. Second, many companies have established special committees to study their particular health care situations. These committees are developing increased knowledge of, and skepticism about, many proposed approaches to cost containment. They particularly want to know whether proposed approaches will really work, and they want long-term results. Third, companies are increasingly willing to intervene directly in the health care system. Instead of passively shuffling dollars to an insurer and then to doctors and hospitals, companies increasingly acknowledge that they are buying health care for their employees and not health insurance protection.

After we began observing these changes, the National Chamber Foundation gave InterStudy the opportunity to respond to them by developing a national health strategy for business. In preparing the five reports that comprise this strategy, InterStudy relied heavily on the input of an outstanding advisory committee made up of leaders from business, insurance, and the health care field. We hope that the series will be the most practical guide available on the subject of how corporations can contain health costs and use their influence to help improve the performance of the health system.

The first report is entitled "How Business Interacts with the Health Care System." It provides quick insight into the unique organizational arrangements and incentives that shape our health system's behavior, and offers specific suggestions on how to evaluate a company's health care experience. For instance, most firms are running around 900 days or more of hospitalization per 1,000 individuals per year. This report points out that you can get just as much health out of the health care system for 650 days of hospitalization. It goes on to identify things like how many admissions or discharges from the hospital you should expect, and so forth.

The role of small business in the health system presents a special problem. Firms with fewer than 500 employees account for approximately half the country's work force of 46 million people. For health insurance purposes, a firm usually needs more than 5,000 employees to be separately experience rated; without this, small businesses are pooled together, which makes it very difficult for a single employer to make an impact on its health care costs. A special section of the first report suggests some ways to get around this problem.

The second report of the series is entitled "How Business Can Use Specific Techniques to Control Health Care Costs." Greater efficiency is often possible in areas like claims processing and payment and coordination of benefits. Once these administrative savings have been realized, most other cost reductions will have to do with the quantity and quality of medical care itself. The report reviews the evidence available on such techniques as second surgical opinions, preadmission certification, and reducing consumer demand by increasing deductibles.

The third report is entitled "How Business Can Stimulate a Competitive Health Care System." The development of a competitive system involves changing the organization and incentives that help shape the health industry. This report focuses on the characteristics and cost-cutting potentials of HMOs and other alternative arrangements for delivering care, which are the key building blocks of any market-oriented health system. All the reports in the series make the general point that the organization and incentives of the health system are responsible for a large part of the cost escalation we are experiencing, and that to control costs we have to give market forces a greater role in medical care.

The fourth report deals with "How Business Can Promote Good Health for Employees and Their Families." This one will perhaps elicit the most interest, particularly from corporate medical departments. The authors present examples of various company health promotion programs and focus on the question of whether they actually work. Since few real cost-benefit studies are available, the report provides a series of descriptions of ways to measure the cost effectiveness of such programs.

The fifth report, "How Business Can Improve Health Planning and Regulation," may be the most controversial of the series and was the most difficult for us to write. We've tried to present a fair evaluation of the regulatory mechanisms for containing costs, describing in detail how the various methods of health planning and regulation are being applied federally, in states, and in communities. Business people are being called upon to staff several hundred HSAs around the country, and indeed, these agencies have little chance of succeeding in containing costs if they continue to be dominated by either the providers of medical care or by the political system. Because of the antiregulatory mood that is sweeping the country and because controls on entry and prices in any industry are anathema to most businesspeople, the report includes a debate on the merits of regulation versus competition in the health care industry. In the absence of significant change in the structure of the health industry, regulation may be the only practical approach to a growing problem. The health system is currently behaving just the way industry is paying it to behave, and if we are not satisfied with the price, quality, and availability of the product, then only industry can do something about it. This series tells how.

Mr. Ozga:

The National Chamber is determined not to let the InterStudy reports be just another nice-looking study that never gets off the shelf. The recommendations included in the reports are sound, practical solutions to problems that bedevil every businessperson in the country. Accordingly, the National Chamber is embarking on a nationwide publicity and community action program to help industry make use of the InterStudy documents.

One of the methods for achieving this objective is to add a manual containing the following components: A chapter entitled "Health Action . . . Why?," which describes the reasons that business and concerned citizens should be involved in improving health and containing costs. A second chapter, called "Health Action . . . How?," explains how to get started and proceed with a successful action program. A third chapter, "Health Action . . . Where?," shows through a case study format how private action is succeeding in improving health and containing costs. The fourth chapter, "Health Action . . . What?," summarizes each of the strategy reports and the action plan suggested. Action teams will find the five strategy reports and this manual to be very useful in planning meetings.

The National Chamber of Commerce is uniquely qualified to make these reports known through its membership of over 80,000, including 2,600 state and local chambers. In addition, we will be utilizing to the fullest extent our broadcasting and printing media, including *Nation's Business*; the November 1978 issue carries a story on our program.

The publicity effort will be supplemented by an active assistance effort. We will be providing first-hand technical assistance to selected localities and chambers of commerce. A special task force has been formed to serve as a speakers' bureau and referral agent to other sources of technical assistance. We are also considering conducting technical assistance seminars at major metropolitan chambers.

Finally, the Chamber's health action program recognizes that there are a variety of reasons for the health care dilemma and all the contributors to this problem—government, doctors, hospitals, insurers, labor, business, and the general public—need to cooperate in finding solutions. To be effective in this effort, employers need to become more knowledgeable about the health care system—to know where the problems are, what causes them, and where they can be most effective in finding solutions. According to the Council on Wage and Price Stability:

> Cost control incentives proposed by the private sector promise to be more effective than those imposed by the multitude of government agencies . . . The private sector is motivated by economic incentives which the government will simply never share . . . [These] incentive[s] . . . [have] been the missing factor[s] in health care . . . the key ingredient[s] in bringing about much needed change in the system . . . In our opinion, the private sector is up to the challenge.

This action program on health is the National Chamber's way of accepting this challenge. Please join us.

Mr. White:

The health insurance industry is generally viewed as ineffective, at best, in controlling health costs. One of our own surveys shows that only 18 percent of the public thinks we are playing a major role in this effort. That is terribly disturbing to us, because nothing could be further from the truth. Insurance companies share the same concern as everybody else with the cost of health care, and when we determined this year to undertake an unprecedented communications program to speak out to the American people on priority health care issues, we knew exactly which priority we wanted to speak about: rising costs.

The communications program was approved early last year by the Health Insurance Association, an organization representing over 300 companies selling health insurance. Responsibility for developing the program's content and strategy was given to the Health Insurance Institute, the public relations organization which I head. We determined that the program should be a total communications effort, combining national advertising and public relations on a scale never before attempted in our business.

Initially, we are concentrating in six promising areas and making each the focus of an ad:

1. The creation of more hospital budget review commissions, such as exist in Maryland, Connecticut, and Massachusetts, which are saving millions of dollars.
2. The adoption of an effective certificate of need program in every state to avoid wasteful duplication of hospital facilities, equipment, and services.
3. A greater self-responsibility for health on the part of the individual.
4. Getting knowledgeable people involved in the health planning process in order to improve and strengthen that process.
5. Stressing alternatives to costly hospital care, such as HMOs, outpatient centers, and so forth.
6. Reducing surgical costs by encouraging second opinions and minor surgery on an outpatient basis.

Two of the ads have already appeared, the first on hospital budget review and the second on certificate of need; the third will appear in the near future. The third conveys that the best way to avoid the high cost of sickness is, very simply, to stay well. The messages that appear over the next year will be carefully tailored to whatever the future environment is.

The first ad had a provocative message. It said that America has a problem that is spreading faster than cancer, heart disease, and hypertension, and the answer on the facing page of the two-page ad is "Costs!" The copy is illustrative of the theme that runs throughout all our messages—that though our health care system is basically sound and though private health insurers have made strides in protecting people against costs, still, no one has done enough.

The advertising is only the beginning. Under the public relations plan we have developed, every participating insurance company has been asked to appoint a so-called program coordinator. We have urged all the insurance trade associations to carry out public relations projects with regard to the advertising theme. Finally, we have within the insurance business a network of state health care committees, each of which has been asked to undertake public relations activities to help spread the word.

To aid all these groups in carrying out such an amibitious undertaking, we provided a lot of material, including something we call an action guide. This book contains a great number of suggestions for public relations projects that can be carried out within the companies and within the communities.

Another dimension to this industry effort reflects the recognition that it is not enough to inform the public about our concern and the solutions we propose. The commitment we express in words must be backed up by a commitment in fact. Insurance companies are doing more than ever to cut costs, but we all recognize the need to do even more. Getting insurance companies involved even more in health care cost containment is a major thrust of this communications program.

One of the ways we prepared for this effort was to survey a number of insurance companies of varying size and location to determine exactly what they were doing in health care cost control. The results of the survey helped us to develop the guidelines in the action guide. Overall, these activities revolve around four major areas: benefit plan design, claims review procedures, educational programs, and support of other voluntary or, where appropriate, mandatory programs.

The efforts require the cooperation of employers and provider groups. The real key to benefit plan design, for example, lies in the acceptance by management and labor of those benefits that maximize incentives for economical care. If hospitals and doctors do not cooperate on pre–hospital admission testing programs or on second surgical opinion programs, we have lost another avenue of cost containment. And obviously, peer review and utilization review will not succeed unless doctors and hospitals cooperate.

Perhaps no trend has captured the interest of so many groups, our own industry included, as programs of prevention and education to improve the health status of employees and their families. I see no reason why more insurance companies and their clients can't cooperate in the development of prevention programs for employees by distributing informational materials, sponsoring physical fitness activities, conducting research on employee health habits, and various other activities.

Finally, it seems to me that there is enormous potential in bringing together leaders in the private sector—business, labor, and the health professions—to give support to model programs in the community that deal with health cost problems. In effect, the private sector should present a united front in attacking the most serious concern we have in health care.

At the same time I have to note that, while our business does support the Voluntary Effort, it also supports appropriate legislative effort to get the job done. We feel that this matter is so serious that all the resources of our country should be brought to bear on the problem. This is why our business is on record as supporting hospital budget review commissions in each state, why we support an effective certificate of need process and a strengthening of the health planning process. But I am convinced that with the joint involvement and support of all of us in the private sector, we will have the weapon to fight health cost inflation.

Mr. Earle:

I want to give you a status report on the VE, speculate a bit on its near-term future, and then offer a few suggestions on how business can help to control health care costs.

The VE began in December 1977 with the formation of the National Steering Committee, whose role is to set policy guidelines and targets for the industry. The expectation is that these guidelines will be met through the vehicle of state-level health cost containment committees. Of course, the real action has to take place on the community level. While the focus is on the hospital, this program is designed to get at all health care cost increases. The National Steering Committee is a broadly based coalition of the key interests in the health care field, including the hospitals, the doctors, the HIAA, Blue Cross, business, consumers, local government, and the Health Industry Manufacturers Association. We have invited AFL-CIO and UAW to sit with us at the national level, but so far we have gotten a negative reply. AFL-CIO has taken a formal position against the VE and recommended to their affiliates that they not participate. However, at last count eighteen of the state-level committees had labor representatives.

At the national level we have an effectively functioning coalition of special interests in the health care field. Last December the Steering Committee set out a fifteen-point program, the most significant item of which was to reduce significantly the rate of increase in health care costs and in hospital costs. To translate that into specifics, we have called for a reduction in hospital costs increases of two percentage points in 1978 and another two percentage points in 1979. Our target for 1978 is 13.6 percent, and for 1979, 11.6 percent, compared with 15.6 percent in 1977. The committee also set the goals on the capital spending, which are: no net increase in hospital beds in 1978 and keeping capital spending in 1978 down to at most 80 percent of the last three years' average. Other points in the fifteen-point program address the other key elements of rising health care costs, such as physician utilization, productivity, the role of insurance companies and coverage through the employer-employee relationship, the role of government, and making regulations cost effective.

At its most recent meeting, the National Steering Committee looked at 1979 goals and objectives and took the following actions: It reaffirmed the whole fifteen-point program that was set out last December. The capital expenditure target was updated so that in 1979 we are again calling for no net increase in hospital beds, and again calling for capital spending in hospitals in 1979 to be pegged at maximum of 80 percent of the capital expenditure in the industry over the last four years. In addition, the committee endorsed the statements of Dr. Tom Nesbitt, the AMA's president, in calling for physicians to voluntarily reduce their fee increases over a period of time to bring them down to the Consumer Price Index.

In the first seven months of 1978, we have seen a 12.8 percent increase in costs. In other words, we have already exceeded by almost 1 percent the target we set for the entire year. The hospital industry is seeing a deceleration that began two years before the VE. It seems clear, therefore, that we will meet our 1978 goal. The Steering Committee carefully assessed whether we should change our goal for 1979. We decided to keep the target at 11.6 percent for 1979, because that will mean bringing the rate of increase in hospital spending down to approximately the rate of increase in total GNP.

Two factors have created this downward trend, despite the upward pressure in general inflation. The first is utilization. Length of stay had leveled off for five or six years in a row at 7.4 days per 1,000, but it has now dropped to 7.2 days per 1,000 and it may go to 7.1. Tightened physician utilization, better utilization review, HMO impact, preadmission testing, and outpatient services are some of the many things that are contributing to a tightened utilization of hospital services. The other key factor in the downward trend is better management, reflected in the fact that the use of personnel in hospitals is not going up as fast as total services.

These factors—not state rate review—have caused the cost deceleration in the industry. The White House and HEW really threw out a "red herring," in my opinion, when they said that the apparent success of the VE and the downward cost trend in the industry are strictly due to state rate review. If you take the ten states that are the tightest in terms of increase and do have budget review or rate review, those states average something like 12.4 percent growth in costs. When you take the ten states that have the lowest rate of increase and don't have rate review, you get an aggregate of about 12.5 percent. If you remove New York from the rate review states, the average of the other nine comes out higher than the ten states that don't have rate review.

The point is not that rate review is bad, good, or indifferent. Rate review has a role to play, but it is not the only answer. If we try to rely on state rate review alone, we will never solve this problem. To back that up, let me point out that states like California, Pennsylvania, Texas, and Ohio contributed just as much toward the downward trend in 1978 as states like Connecticut, Maryland, and the others with rate review. In studying the Indiana system, which is a quasi-voluntary rate review system, the conclusion emerges that the single most important factor in Indiana's success is the professional management incentives built into their program. It is not the financial control incentive. That's what we're trying to get through the VE.

Where are we going from here? Next year is going to be tougher, which is another reason why the Steering Committee decided not to change the target for 1979. Double-digit inflation is approaching in the whole economy. Hospitals are heavy users of labor, energy, and food, and all these factors are likely to have high inflation. The lower we get, the tougher it's going to become. There's not that much more you can cut or postpone. The Steering Committee has charged the staff of the VE with assessing what measures would be appropriate beyond 1979. Once we get through next year we will be in a good position to, in effect, set an economic policy for the industry.

Finally, what's the role of business in this effort? It is critical to make this program succeed and business can make the difference. We need business at the national level to help in the policymaking for this industry and to participate in the setting of targets and guidelines, not just for 1979, but beyond. Business should also support and participate in the state and local programs. At the hospital and community level, business can play a key role as members of hospital boards, making sure that each institution's medical staff and management are doing everything they can, and also through participating and providing leadership in the planning process.

I would point out, in addition, that health insurance premium increases ought to be lower than in the past. The hospital industry's downward trend should show up in your premiums. If it doesn't, make your carrier prove the reasonableness of the premiums he's suggesting. You should also be looking at the HMO option, looking at self-insurance, looking at other ways to reduce that premium dollar and to put pressure on the marketplace. Industry is in the position to do it because industry is the big buyer.

Question Period

Willis Goldbeck, WBGH: Dr. Ellwood, would you comment on the potential of the VE?

Dr. Ellwood: The VE will only work if it can restructure the incentives in the industry. We're not seeing a downward curve right now, but rather a slight flattening of the curve; and I don't think that even that will persist without basic changes in the system. The reason we have this problem in the first place is that this industry is behaving just the way you have rewarded it to behave. The VE is beginning to get at basic changes.

Let me comment on the role the private sector can play, versus the government. Only you really have the kinds of incentives that will change behavior to result in changes in the health system. The government doesn't. The government tries to control people's behavior through laws and regulations, and I can tell you as a physician that we can beat the government every time. Unless you are ready to change the rules that we play by, the incentives in our business, we'll beat you every time. Business shouldn't necessarily accept the health industry's guidelines. There is no reason why inflation in health care should remain higher than inflation in the general economy, and business should work to bring it down.

Neils Nielsen, ARA Services: Why doesn't there seem to be any evidence of improved productivity as a result of the investment in new technology in health care?

Dr. Ellwood: Unfortunately, technology in this field at this time tends to be additive instead of substitutive. Until you change our incentives so that we can gain by saving money rather than by adding to costs, then we are going to see costs rise. You've got to put us into a position where we've got to deliver more for less, and I'll bet you we can. It's startling how good physicians can be at containing costs when you put us in a position where we have to do it, and how different an approach we take from the regulators. When physicians have to contain costs, they go after quantity and content of care. When regulators have to contain costs, they go after supply of resources and prices. If you want us to deliver the product better and cheaper, then direct more business toward those providers who provide you more for less.

Samuel Howard, Hospital Affiliates International: How can inflation ever be brought under control as long as the government, which accounts for 40 percent of health expenditures, continues to use cost-based reimbursement?

Dr. Ellwood: Some change will definitely be needed. However, it will probably only occur after the private sector demonstrates that it can control costs by using other reimbursement systems.

Philip Lescohier, International Harvester: Why has the VE opposed the Nelson cost containment proposal, which would only have gone into effect if the VE failed?

Mr. Earle: The VE itself did not take a position. The AMA, AHA, and FAH opposed it for two reasons. One was that the controls that would have been triggered were formulistic and applied across the board. Thus, they would not take into account the differing circumstances at different hospitals. The other reason was that they believe that stand-by controls are inherently inflationary and become a self-fulfilling prophecy.

Diana Walsh, Center for Industry and Health Care: Is the threat of antitrust impeding the efforts of the insurance industry or the VE to contain costs?

Mr. White: One of the reasons that the Health Insurance Institute is limiting itself to a public communications effort is that more substantive collaborative efforts might invite antitrust enforcement.

Mr. Earle: We have taken steps to minimize antitrust issues in our program at all levels.

William McHenry, Coopers & Lybrand: Are any of the cost containment programs used by business particularly widespread or effective?

Dr. Ellwood: We have found no pattern in the use of programs; nor were the data good enough in many locations to determine the effectiveness of any given program. In the long run, however, the diversity in approaches should lead to a few effective programs that can be replicated by other businesses.

Michael Riley, AMA: Senator Kennedy is using examples of people who were financially ruined by a catastrophic illness to push his national health insurance proposal. Is the insurance industry pushing catastrophic coverage, since this might blunt the drive for NHI?

Mr. White: Our estimate is that 150 million people now have catastrophic coverage. It is a rapidly expanding coverage and the companies are marketing it aggressively.

Dr. Ellwood: While this is probably the most important social issue in health, it is also the most difficult area in which to contain costs. The proportion of high-cost episodes is growing, and that poses a major threat to any cost control effort.

COMMENTARY

Richard E. Emrick, Director, Benefit Programs, Mead Corporation

All the private sector cost control efforts presented by this panel are quite laudatory and appear on the surface to have considerable merit. However, they all assume that business, providers, and users of the health care system will have totally redirected drives and attitudes as a result of these activities. I tend to believe this is idealistic and naive.

What we are facing in the health care industry and with the people using it is an evolved societal philosophy that says:

1. My existence warrants certain care and treatment without any inconvenience or difficult decisions on my part.
2. Life is important and no cost limitations should apply to the treatment of my family and me when we are sick or injured.
3. "Good" health insurance should cover all such costs with minimal outlay, if any, on my part.
4. Users want the best health care, and as physicians and hospitals, we will meet their wants without too much concern about costs.

I have serious trouble believing that any of these private initiatives will really succeed because those who helped create current attitudes are those who are being called upon to carry the burden of change. The suggested approaches do not provide a program to remold the general attitude of society.

The business community is placed in an untenable position as well. Despite the recently invoked voluntary wage and price limits, businesses have been raising their prices, presumably to the extent the market, if any, will bear. How can business easily turn and point the finger at another sector (the physicians and hospitals) without some reservations?

Intervention by business cannot and will not be uniform enough to make a big difference in the short term. Major businesses will try to use parts of these proposed programs, but they have bottom lines to be concerned about. Allocations of personnel time and money for a very uncertain return won't be made very easily. Moreover, the many small businesses in the United States just don't have the capability of taking the suggested actions, including front money to finance alternate delivery systems.

The unions have a totally different attitude. Led by the UAW with its bent for more and more first-dollar coverage, they are just not going to be able to switch direction with their membership, even if they believed that a change in direction was warranted. The Kennedy NHI bill is being pushed because it preserves what the union has won and includes proposed cost controls, which might have as "good" a chance of working as anything else. Business management is not likely to endure prolonged strikes to secure a change away from first-dollar coverage. Unions don't want to change the public attitude.

The insurers (commercial and Blue Cross–Blue Shield) have even less credibility with their business activities. Blue Cross–Blue Shield spearheaded (with union endorsement) the move to semiprivate and UCRO first-dollar coverage. To protect their market share, the commercial insurers have joined the bandwagon. Since 1974, yearly group insurance contract renewals have involved substantial increases. The insurance industry knew what was happening but never stepped forward very strongly to intervene. Only after major employers forced them to accept revised underwriting approaches (minimum premium and ASO) for cost savings did they react. Raising the flag now to charge against costs is just acting too late in the game. Their tarnished image, whether imagined or real, will impede the effectiveness of their activities. They represent too loose a coalition to be effective in changing public attitudes.

What about the providers themselves and their voluntary efforts? They are in much the same posture as the insurance industry. While they do have strong associations, their associations are trying to leverage a large number of independent business units through state and local medical societies. We all hope that the VE will work, but the outcome is very questionable.

A change in the public's attitude toward its rights and obligations in our society has to begin in Washington, D.C. If the federal government through its programs continues to promise something to everyone without cost consequences, there will be no basis for an attitudinal change that will permit any voluntary effort to succeed. It may well be too late.

Labor Looks at National Health Insurance

Cramer M. Gilmore II, Max W. Fine, and Bert Seidman

Mr. Gilmore: I would like to tell you briefly the Teamsters' position on NHI by reading from a resolution that was passed June 14, 1976 at our convention in Las Vegas.

> "Whereas the cost of health care has soared to unprecedented heights with no reversal of the upward trend in sight, and, whereas the American people are spending more than the people of any other nation for health care purposes, and whereas no other national health insurance bill includes mechanisms to control costs at the source, preserve quality care and place the emphasis on patients and their needs, rather than insurance companies, hospitals, and doctors; therefore be it resolved that we petition the Congress and the candidates for President of the United States to publicly and explicitly endorse the National Health Security Act, known as the Kennedy-Corman Bill, to guarantee that every American has quality health care at a cost that he or she can afford."

Since 1960, the per capita personal health care expenditures in the United States have gone up about 500 percent and, during the period—1970–1977 they have gone up approximately 280 percent. You can readily understand why the Teamsters are so concerned at the bargaining table about the level of benefits that they can afford and, more particularly, about maintaining the noncontributory status of those benefits.

The Council on Employee Benefits has predicted that by the late 1980s the percentage of payroll that will be spent for fringe benefits will be in the magnitude of 55 percent, and I think it is worth looking at how they break that down. The Council surveyed 101 companies, and 76 responded with their views on what benefits they expect to be fairly widespread in the middle of the 1980s. The benefits include expanded dental coverage, additional vacation in the first year of employment, and statements of the costs of the benefits. Commonly expected between 1980 and 1985 were free retirement counseling, second-opinion surgery, "stop-loss" provisions to put a limitation on out-of-pocket expenses, nursing home coverage, additional fixed holidays, "flex" time, a shorter work week, more vacation, and an additional floating holiday.

A very large gap exists between the expectations of companies regarding increased health care benefits (expanded dental coverage, second opinion surgery, and stop-loss provisions) and the reality of negotiations in 1978 for health care benefits. The facts are that workers' out-of-pocket expenses are growing because of increased deductible amounts, higher rates of coinsurance, and fee-for-service schedules that are so badly outdated that the workers' share of coinsurance is approaching the insurance fee in many cases. In reality, the workers' share of health care costs is growing as well as the employers' share. This is a very serious and debilitating problem for organized labor whose members are alarmingly threatened by inflation in general and health care cost inflation in particular.

What has happened in the health care industry that makes health costs out strip the consumer price index in recent years by approximately 100 percent? Clearly there is no obvious answer to this extremely complex and perplexing question. However, the many component parts of health care give some indication of why costs have risen so dramatically. The sudden surge of medical malpractice litigation in this decade has added untold millions—perhaps billions—of dollars to physicians' fees. As a result of the increased incidence of malpractice litigation, "defensive medicine"—precautionary screening procedures and oftentimes duplicated diagnostic procedures—has contributed to hospital charges and physicians' fees which are also escalating at an alarming rate.

The number of hospital beds per 1,000 persons continued to increase in this decade despite economics which suggested that consumption of hospital room and board costs would probably not match this increase. Some health planners have openly spoken out against greater hospital capacity because of the adverse cost consequences of under-utilization which has exacerbated the room and board charges.

Another factor contributing to health care cost increases has been the persistent demand and production of high-technology, high-cost medical equipment. Neurosurgery and cardiopulmonary procedures have made quantum leaps in available services which improve health care while the costs associated with these additional services have also experienced quantum increases. CAT scanners, "coronary by-pass" heart surgery, and sophisticated heart monitors have improved medical science and health care dramatically as well as increasing the costs associated with these two areas of health care.

The overall use of improved medical technologies must be continually reviewed with respect to achievement of better health care. For example, some physicians maintain that increased use of the fetal monitor has not necessarily improved the infant survival rate and, in some cases, may have been inappropriate under certain circumstances. The fetal monitor has, however, contributed to improved care under many delivery circumstances.

Unnecessary surgery, including discretionary and cosmetic surgery, has also contributed to higher health care costs which have approximately doubled the inflation rate of the consumer price index. Without making reference to hard data which may be available, for example, on coronary by-pass survery, the long-term effects of this costly procedure may show less desirable data than the current number of procedures justifies.

The question that we, as members of organized labor must ask ourselves is, are the working people of this country who have contributed to its greatness, to its industrial power, and to corporate profits which have financed more growth and an increasingly affluent society—entitled to basic health care so they can continue to help America grow? Who in good conscience could say no to this question?

Yet we have seen the standard of living of our country's coal miners and their families threatened by a cutback of health and welfare benefits and a greater share of the cost of their remaining benefits. And this loss of workers' real income in recent years owing to escalating health care costs has occured in the same decade in which wages were held to 5.5 percent for a period of time when the cost of medical services was nearly three times the rate of wage increases. The bottom line of runaway medical costs is painfully obvious to us: health care costs in this country are seriously undermining the standard of living of millions of America's working people.

The thrust of recent major contract negotiations regarding health and welfare benefits is no longer concerned with major improvements in benefits, but instead is trying desperately to maintain existing benefits. Maintenance of benefits clauses or "MOB" are a relatively recent phenomenon in health and welfare bargaining and have appeared largely in response to premium levels which are not sufficient to maintain a level of benefits in the face of soaring costs. And workers are paying more out of pocket, not less.

What is the answer to this terrible dilemma that is threatening the very fiber of America—our family welfare? National health insurance to maintain the well-being of our members; NHI to stabilize needlessly soaring health costs; NHI to stop the erosion of workers' purchasing power; NHI to provide health care as a right of every person in this country and not only those who can afford to pay any price for good health. Teamsters General President Fitzsimmons and General Secretary Treasurer Schoessling are members of the Committee of 100 for national health insurance and are actively involved in this major objective of organized labor. The Teamsters are concerned about the growing need for NHI because of the spiraling costs of health care and the erosion of our members standard of living which is largely effected by health care cost inflation. We support the principle of national health care as a right of every working man and woman in this country and we feel that unprecedented increases in medical care costs have brought this concept to the brink of necessity.

Mr. Fine:

You are probably aware that Theodore Roosevelt during the 1912 Bull Moose campaign was the first president to propose NHI. Woodrow Wilson proposed it again in 1916, but the next year the United States got into the First World War, and it was shelved. In 1920 it was revived, but the American Medical Association called it Bolshevism. It was effectively dead for fourteen years, when FDR brought the Committee for Economic Security to Washington in 1934. That was the group that developed the original Social Security Act over the next year, and part of the original proposal to FDR was NHI along with the Old Age Pension plan. Dr. Ross McIntire, sent to see the President by the AMA, said, "If you don't pull that out of the package, we're going to campaign across this country against the Old Age Pension program and against the Social Security program." And FDR said, "Well, we'll take it out, and we'll study it," and they proceeded with the Social Security Act.

NHI was introduced again by Senator Wagner prior to the Second World War, and during that war the War Labor Board froze wages but permitted fringe benefits to be subject to negotiation. That was really the genesis of private health insurance in this country.

Right after the war, after most of the industrial countries in the world began adopting NHI or national health service programs, President Truman sent up as the first domestic message a proposal for a national health program. The only piece of that that was adopted was the Hill-Burton Act, which was very significant. The AMA hired a public relations firm which spent at least $10 million. They created those scare words, "socialized medicine," which they still use to great effect.

When Eisenhower became president, he denied the need for NHI. Later, however, in the summer of 1954, he did perceive a problem that many millions of people could not get private coverage because of preexisting conditions or other reasons, and he proposed a federal revolving fund of $25 billion to bail out the insurance companies if they would provide coverage for the people who were poor risks. The AMA called that "socialized medicine" and that was dead. A year or two later the people who had been involved with President Truman's effort began the push for Medicare. That took eight or nine years to pass and we all know that it was called "socialized medicine."

After the enactment of Medicare, the late Walter Reuther began to plan the effort that resulted in the formation of the Committee for National Health Insurance in late 1968, along with the AFL-CIO, the Teamsters, and the Committee of 100. We developed over eighteen months the original Kennedy-Griffith Bill, and then the Kennedy-Corman Bill. Of course, these were opposed by Presidents Nixon and Ford and the business community on the basis of the huge shift of private funds onto the public budget. During the 1976 campaign, Jimmy Carter made a specific commitment to the principles in the Kennedy-Corman Bill, and they were adopted at Carter's request by the Democratic Platform Committee.

We worked alongside the administration in the last year and a half to try to develop a feasible bill. The President laid down two constraints: minimal impact on the federal budget and a significant role for the private insurance companies. After a great deal of work we believed we had fashioned a bill that was responsive to his constraints and yet forsook none of the basic principles of the Health Security Bill, which were, first and foremost, that health care should be a matter of right. Yet after reaching this point in our discussions with the White House and HEW, we found a new constraint. The program would be phased in over a period of years, but each phase would be triggered by another Congress, perhaps, and perhaps phased in only if extraneous issues such as the economy permitted. That caused the breakdown of the discussions because that was at variance with the basic principle of health care as a right and not something tied to a condition.

Senator Kennedy proceeded, along with Mr. Meany, Doug Frazier, and all the others who support our approach, to announce the preliminary plan that we now call the Health Care for All Americans Act of 1979. There is a tremendous amount of work to do in fashioning a bill out of this preliminary plan, but it does provide for everyone to be covered, for employers to provide benefits for employees and contribute at least 75 percent of the premium cost, and for the federal government to finance the benefits for the elderly as part of an expanded Medicare program, for the poor, and for the unemployed.

It provides for immediate cost controls upon enactment, with the benefits to begin two years later, so we don't repeat the mistakes of Medicare. It provides, following the start of benefits, a budgeting system much like that in Canada for hospital and physicians' fees. For the first time, what fee is reasonable will be determined through the process of negotiation, and not arbitrarily set. It provides for a public authority to be selected by the President and approved by the Senate to oversee the program. It provides for the delegation of authority to the states in terms of assuring that the budgeting process is carried out and representing the public interests at the state level. It provides that the people would have a choice, much like the one federal employees have today, among a consortium, which Ætna represents in the federal program, Blue Cross–Blue Shield, or an HMO.

Everybody would have a health insurance card and it would not be identifiable in terms of the financing, so that we wouldn't have a two-class system. Even if you didn't have a card and you showed up at the hospital and received the medical care you needed, the hospital would be paid. The state authority would determine who was responsible for the payment, whether it was Consortium A, Consortium B, the HMO, or the federal government.

It provides for federal regulation of the health insurance carriers. It provides for quality control incentives for HMOs, competition among the carriers, a reinsurance fund to take care of catastrophic risks, maintenance of existing employee-employer relationships, and so forth.

We urge you as members of the business community not to discard this proposal the way the AMA did two weeks ago when Senator Kennedy began his public hearings on it. They took the old script that they had used for years against the Health Security Act and simply presented that as testimony.

We urge you to familiarize yourself with this plan, to testify about it, to help fashion it because it's not cast in concrete. Labor and management can never begrudge fine quality medical care, but maybe it's time that we together took a much sharper look at what we're buying. I doubt that there is anything that American industry buys over which it has less control as to cost or quality than medical care. We face a very trying period in the next year in negotiating contracts. The increased cost of health care could consume a major portion of the 7 percent lid on increases. We used to think that there was something more important to industry than its own self-interest when it rejected the Health Security Bill, and that was concern about shifting billions of dollars onto the federal budget. Well, we're not talking about that kind of program anymore and we think that it's in the self-interest of industry as well as in the public interest that you seriously consider supporting the current approach that's in this new plan.

Mr. Seidman:

A labor-management group, composed of some of the top management and labor representatives in the country and assisted by a technical task force, has developed a series of recommendations in the health care field. These were issued as the "Labor-Management Group Position Papers on Health Care Costs." I served on that task force as cochairman on the labor side.

It pleased me very much that we found a remarkable degree of agreement on goals in the health care field between the labor and management representatives, both at the policy level and at the technical level. Such goals as reducing health care costs, developing a more rational and efficient health care system, improving the quality of care, and taking steps to ensure a more effective role for labor and management in the development of health care policy were shared by both sides.

This agreement wasn't limited just to broad goals. We also found that we could agree in many specific ways on methods of achieving those goals—on prospective reimbursement, development of HMOs, health planning, hospital preadmission testing, prospective surgical review, utilization review of hospital services, the expansion of alternatives to inpatient hospital treatment, the role of nurse practitioners and physician assistants in controlling health care costs, the impact of medical technology on hospital costs, the problems arising with respect to medical malpractice, and the need for health education. And under each of those headings, we could agree on a broad range of recommendations.

However, in failing to come to grips with the need for NHI, management is acting against its own interests. While it is true that some of the goals sought in the Labor-Management Group Position Papers can, to a greater or lesser degree, be achieved without NHI, those goals will be achieved sooner and more effectively in an NHI framework. Second, without the key features of NHI, we are not going to be able to achieve effective and lasting control of health care costs.

Let me try to dispel an illusion that some people may have. Some believe that you can reduce health care costs by passing them on to the workers, perhaps by changing a noncontributory plan to a contributory plan, or by requiring deductibles and co-insurance where they don't exist, or by enlarging deductibles and co-insurance where they are already in place. But the workers and their families, unless they are covered for comprehensive care in an HMO, are already paying out of pocket upwards of 50 percent of their health care costs. Organized labor has been for first-dollar coverage for a long time, and we don't intend to change our position on that. Organized labor will not buy the take-away idea because workers won't put up with it, and if you don't believe me, all you have to do is look at the experience of the Mine Workers and the Auto Workers and all the rest.

These are the essential principles of NHI that organized labor has consistently supported: a comprehensive single standard of benefits—that means no second-class citizens, health care as a right, universal coverage, reform of the delivery system, built-in quality control, effective cost control, and minimal administrative overhead costs. We are paying in this country 13–20 percent of health care costs for administrative costs, while in Canada, with universal comprehensive NHI, they are paying about 2.5 percent. And we have one more essential principle: that the program must be phased in through a fixed timetable, laid out in a single piece of legislation.

Let me zero in again on the main cost control features of our plan. We agree with the administration on hospital cost control. But it's the physicians who control health care costs; it's what they do or don't do that determines what health care costs are going to be. It is essential, therefore, that there be negotiation with physician representatives over fair fee schedules—fair to them and fair to the rest of the country—and that the physicians then be held to these schedules.

Unlike the Kennedy-Corman Bill, the new Kennedy proposal does provide a role for the insurance industry. I don't think that was necessary in terms of the intrinsic problems that we face, but the people who have been working for NHI during the past decade have come to the conclusion that it is necessary to provide a role for private insurance if we are going to get a plan enacted.

But the insurance industry in this country has been part of the problem and not part of the solution. It hasn't been taking the initiative, until very recently, and then only in full-page ads. And so, while this bill provides a role for private insurance, it also provides for strict control of the private insurance industry.

It provides for the development of HMOs and for other organized settings for the delivery of care. If you cut the cost of hospitalization in half, as HMOs do, that's going to do a lot to control the cost of medical care. And the plan provides a strong and effective role for consumers.

Let me say something about the role of management in this connection. As purchasers of medical care, you are consumers, and your interests lie not with the providers of medical care, not with the AMA and AHA and the health insurance industry, but with organized labor and other consumer groups concerned about the cost and quality of care. Participation in preparing the "Labor-Management Group Position Papers on Health Care Costs" has demonstrated that management is not afraid of advancing and promoting its interests and its concerns in the health care field, but I think that this is only a first step. Those who will resist all efforts to control runaway cost escalation are already organized to fight every inch of the way against any legislation, whether it be cost control legislation or NHI legislation. They are girding their loins to stave off any NHI, and if they can't kill it outright, they'll try to make sure that it does not have the kinds of provisions that make possible the handle on health care costs that you want and we all need.

You do have an alternative. You can join with us in supporting a universal, comprehensive NHI program with effective and equitable cost controls. I hope you feel as we do that, at long last, health care should be the right of every American. But, whether or not you adhere to that fundamental principle, I know you share our desire to stop the uncontrolled escalation of health care costs, and there is only one way to do that: enactment at the earliest possible date of universal, comprehensive NHI. Labor and management and the whole country can no longer afford not to have it.

Question Period

Freddie Lucas, General Motors: How could the proposed fixed timetable for phasing in the plan take into account future conditions?

Mr. Seidman: We want to avoid having political battles on this issue over and over again. Therefore, we want to have the program introduced in a single piece of legislation with a fixed timetable for the introduction of whatever phases or stages may be necessary. It will always be possible for a future Congress at any time to repeal the legislation. We want to put the burden on those who want to hold back the program to prove that restraint is necessary.

Willis Goldbeck, WBGH: Could we have a clarification of the proposed earnings-based premium and how it would differ from a tax?

Mr. Seidman: The premium would be paid either to Blue Cross–Blue Shield or to an insurance company. This same feature is contained in a number of other proposals; it would require employers to pay on behalf of their employees and would permit a 75–25 percent sharing of the cost. As far as the earnings-based premium is concerned, it is our feeling that it would be most equitable to make the amount of the premium relate to the amount of wages. Otherwise, it would be regressive financing.

William McHenry, Coopers & Lybrand: What would be the role of the federal public authority under the new plan?

Mr. Fine: The public authority under the present bill would be appointed by the President with the concurrence of the Senate, and it would have responsibility for carrying out public aspects of the program. The public aspects would include federal regulation of the health insurance carriers, although actual administration would be carried out largely by the members of the three consortia—the commercial companies, the Blues, and the HMOs—under state authorities, to whom the federal authority would delegate powers, both in terms of the health aspects and the insurance regulatory aspects.

Frank Finkenberg, George B. Buck Consulting Actuaries: Would there be any place for self-insured employer plans or self-insured joint labor-management trust plans in the proposal?

Mssrs. Fine and Seidman: We expect that there would be, although the details have not yet been worked out.

Richard Egdahl, Center for Industry and Health Care: Is there any role for a pure private sector completely outside the national plan?

Mr. Seidman: There probably would be such a system, but few people would use it. The experience in Canada is that 2 or 3 percent of the people buy services outside the system.

Mr. Goldbeck: What is labor's view of some current cost-control efforts, such as the VE?

Mr. Seidman: I support a wage passthrough under any cost containment plan. I have reviewed the budgets for the community hospitals in Fairfax County, Virginia, where I reside, and the hospitals were very proud that they were going to hold to the voluntary guidelines by holding their increase to only 11 percent next year. And how were they going to do that? By holding the wages of their unorganized hospital workers to 5 percent. Well, we don't want any of that.

Mr. Gilmore: The Teamsters represent a substantial number of hospital workers, typically orderlies, guards, cooks, and so on, and their wages are notoriously low. I am sure they are lower on average than other public employees get in similar classifications. So when one talks about cost containment in hospitals, it really strikes a nerve that labor could end up with the short end of the stick. This is not the way organized labor would like to see cost containment realized.

Ronald Hurst, Caterpillar Tractor: What is your view of IPA-type HMOs?

Mr. Seidman: I think IPAs are better than nothing, and they will be more effective in areas where there are one or more prepaid group practice plans. In the first place, I think that group practice, in and of itself, is a more effective and efficient way of providing medical care. In addition to that, it is very much more difficult for the IPAs to control what their individual doctor-members do. The doctors in an IPA are paid on a fee-for-service basis, and they have all the perverse incentives of the fee-for-service system. The only control is that the people who are covered by the program are paying on a capitation basis. Therefore, IPAs know that their income is limited. The experience of IPAs is that they have not been able to reduce, for example, the hospitalization rate as much as have prepaid group practice plans, except in an area like St. Paul, where the IPA has had to exercise very considerable amounts of discipline on its doctor-members because of the competition of prepaid group practice plans.

COMMENTARY

Samuel H. Howard, Vice-President, Planning, Hospital Affiliates International, Inc.

Historically, large industrial labor unions, the CIO, and later the United Auto Workers have spearheaded the recurrent demands for NHI. More recently, their special aim has been to eliminate health insurance costs, generally the most expensive fringe benefit, from contract negotiations with management. With the inauguration of President Carter, NHI again became prominent on the governmental agenda, and Senator Kennedy, its leading congressional proponent, has recently issued the outline of a revised proposal.

In national opinion surveys conducted in the early 1970s, a majority of Americans agreed that there was a crisis in health care. However, as it related to them personally, they did not appear to be too concerned. What dominates the crisis conception of American medicine in congressional committees is the problem of medical costs, as expressed in the testimony of government program managers, insurance company executives, and union leaders. The various other "problems" mentioned are simply defects that any sensible analyst would identify, not conditions uniformly worsening so as to justify predictions of disaster.

The concern about rapidly rising health care costs is a valid one. However, this concern should not be addressed by implementing a comprehensive NHI program—at least, not one that calls for first-dollar coverage and a major role for the federal government in the financing and delivery of health care. Our appetite for medical care appears to be nearly insatiable when it is fully prepaid. Such an NHI program would exacerbate the problem of rapidly rising health care costs.

Increases in health expenditures are caused by a number of factors—some unique to the health industry. Most result from inflation; the rest from changes in the size and age of our population, changes in the kinds of services provided, and changes in utilization. Three features of the health care system make it particularly prone to cost increases. First, health care is somewhat immune to the influence of supply and demand because the decision to purchase a service is made by the physician and not the consumer. Second, medical bills are in large measure paid by third parties. The existence of Medicare, Medicaid, and private insurance plans with low deductibles and little or no coinsurance has dislocated the cost constraint on consumer demand and encouraged consumers to select the "best" and most expensive care available. Further, since health insurance premiums are not included in taxable income, there is an incentive for benefit plans to include more comprehensive coverage.

Modifying the health care system to make use of competition and provide incentives for efficiency would alleviate many of these problems. The greater use of cost sharing (deductibles and co-insurance) in insurance plans would encourage cost-conscious behavior on the part of consumers. The unrestrained development of alternative delivery systems, like HMOs, would bring competition into health care. The replacement of the cost-based system of reimbursing hospitals with a market-oriented financing mechanism would reward the efficient and penalize the inefficient providers.

There remain the problems of the uncovered population and the costs of catastrophic illness. Various estimates of the percentage of the American population without health insurance range from 5 to 10 percent—representing some 10 to 20 million Americans. Most of them cannot afford private coverage but earn too much to qualify for public assistance.

While the number of Americans without health insurance is a large number (whether it be 10 or 20 million), it is important to remember that they represent a small percentage (5–10 percent) of our total population. As former Assistant Secretary of Health Charles E. Edwards states, "It's critical to ask if a mandatory program involving more than 200 million people and drastically changing our entire health care system—one that, although flawed, still delivers the finest medical care to be found anywhere in the world—is the most appropriate remedy for the situation."

Assistance can be extended to the uncovered population through our current programs, subsequent to the implementation of the changes indicated above. The existing health care delivery system need not be reorganized in any fundamental way in order to offer assistance to this part of the population.

According to the Health Insurance Association of America, over 144 million persons—3 out of 4 Americans under age 65—were protected by some form of catastrophic private health insurance in 1976. The number covered by private health insurance is increasing annually as more and more employers offer catastrophic health insurance as an employee benefit. For those persons who are below the poverty line without catastrophic coverage, the answer lies in modifying the Medicaid program.

Indeed, problems of access to adequate medical care, of the uncovered population, and of the lack of coverage for catastrophic illness can be ameliorated by modifications to the existing Medicaid program and by time. Thus, while NHI may have been an appropriate goal during the first half of the century, a comprehensive program is not an appropriate goal today.

If we accept the current estimate of insurance coverage, there exists no pressing need to enact health care legislation providing for "cradle-to-grave," comprehensive health care covering the entire population and providing for unimpeded utilization of the total array of health services. The desire to eliminate health insurance costs from labor contract negotiations is insufficient justification for the federal enactment of a program with many unknown consequences. The implementation of an NHI plan, whether phased or not, could commit the nation to errors of a disastrous magnitude. Uncontrolled escalation of costs, an insupportable level of expenditures, intolerable controls on medical practice, and deterioration in the quality of health services are some of the potential dangers.

COMMENTARY

W. Gordon Binns, Jr., Assistant Treasurer, General Motors Corporation

I have worked closely with Bert on the Labor-Management

Group (LMG) Task Force on Health Care Costs, and I agree with him that this was a very constructive effort. The staff representatives from labor and management saw eye to eye on many important issues, such as the importance of health planning and health education. There was also a general agreement on goals—to issue practical recommendations which, when followed, could help contain health care costs in a variety of ways. The LMG "Position Papers" will be a valuable tool to everyone concerned with controlling health care costs without diminishing the quality of care. Businesspeople are continuing to use and distribute the booklet, just as the labor people are doing.

I also agree with Bert's statement that many of the goals cited in the LMG booklet can be achieved without an NHI program. If labor and management—and doctors and hospitals as well—continue to be responsive to the problem of costs, we can have a positive impact on the health care delivery system.

One of the areas where management and labor did not agree was cost sharing. It seemed to me that most of the audience, in fact, disagreed with Bert's contention that cost sharing is a "take-away" item. Even though it is difficult to measure the extent to which employee cost sharing may reduce health care costs, there is evidence that the person who pays out of pocket for some of the medical services he receives is more likely to question the number of services prescribed, the exact procedures suggested, and the costs of all these. In contrast, the person who pays nothing toward his medical care, and in many cases accepts all services offered without questioning cost, can only serve to run up the aggregate health care bill. Furthermore, employee cost sharing need not create a financial barrier to necessary medical services. Arrangements can certainly be designed that will avoid financial hardship—or even significant burden—on consumers and yet make them more cost conscious than they are in our existing system. There should at least be mutual, objective exploration of the question rather than quick and final dismissal of it as a "take-away."

Although Bert's statement that "the physicians determine what health care costs are going to be" is essentially correct, this very statement suggests that health care costs could be better contained if employees were knowledgeable about the costs of their health care, were motivated to contain these costs, and acted as responsible consumers when dealing with physicians. Well-designed cost sharing could be one way of accomplishing this objective.

I am in agreement with Bert that it should be a national objective that all people have access to adequate health care at an affordable cost, if we can come to an agreement on what that really means. I believe that most of the business community would support this objective. However, the question is not whether this is a laudable objective, but rather how the objective should be achieved. This is where many in the business community disagree with the approach taken by many labor people—radical change in the existing system to arrive at a comprehensive NHI system. It is possible for this objective to be met within the framework of the current health care delivery system. With the cooperation of the insurance carriers, the providers, and labor and management, access to adequate health care for all at an affordable cost can be assured.

I also agree with Bert that management, as a purchaser of medical care, is a "consumer." Our interests lie basically with other consumers, but this is not to say that these interests are opposed to those of the providers. In fact, on most issues involving health care protection for our people, the interests of all involved are much the same. We are working and plan to continue to work with all those involved in the problem of the spiraling costs of health care. Management is involved in many cost containment activities, many in close cooperation with labor. Just one example of this cooperation is the establishment of the Health Alliance Plan, an HMO begun in Detroit through a merger of an already existing HMO with certain facilities of Henry Ford Hospital. This HMO has come into being through the joint efforts of the UAW, Ford, Chrysler, General Motors, and a number of other Detroit employers. The union and the auto companies are all working together on this because all believe that HMOs can be effective at cost containment while providing excellent health care.

As another example, the UAW and General Motors have developed a series of pilot programs to determine whether certain measures are truly effective in containing health care costs. These programs include hospital preadmission testing, presurgical screening, and concurrent utilization review. It is too soon to tell how cost effective these projects will prove to be. However, we will continue to explore all programs that may help contain costs, and will try, in conjunction with the UAW and other unions, to implement any such programs that we may jointly deem desirable.

It is unlikely that labor and management will agree totally on all approaches to health care cost containment. But it is important that we continue to work together toward our mutual objective—to improve the current health care delivery system and make it cost effective.

Public and Private
Together at the Local Level

Industry in Local Health Planning

John Brown, Ronald A. Hurst, and Harry P. Cain, Jr.

Mr. Brown: Genesco's involvement in health planning is perhaps best illustrated by a trip I took recently. A senior vice-president from Blue Cross–Blue Shield of Tennessee picked me up at 8:30 A.M., and we drove to a small community hospital in a rural area. We were going because this hospital has the worst loss ratio of any hospital Genesco deals with. Our plan in this particular town has 270 contracts, and yet this little 32-bed hospital was dispensing close to half a million dollars a year in services to Genesco employees. Last year the claims paid versus premiums collected for our plant in this county was a net loss in excess of $100,000, and experience so far indicated that the loss for this year would exceed $350,000. I was very anxious to see this facility because it was wrecking the experience of our health care program for this particular operating company. We pulled into town, went to the plant and picked up our plant manager and personnel director, and proceeded on to a meeting with the hospital director and the Board of Trustees.

The trip really began three years ago, when I first learned about HSAs and began participating in the health planning process. In the first meeting that I attended of the Middle Tennessee HSA, there was no question that the provider community dominated the HSA itself, the Projects Review Committee, and the Executive Committee. I made application for the Board of Directors and spent almost a year to gain election. I had been told by very knowledgeable providers that the only way that Genesco could truly influence the health care system was to get on the inside, understand how it functions, and be able to identify the pressure points.

The greatest pressure point is knowledge of the system and knowing what questions to ask. The answers, for the most part, are not even available at this time. One of the things I found out early on was that Genesco did not have adequate information with which to manage our health care programs.

Starting early in 1975, we began developing a data system that would help provide the information we needed. Our system enabled us to identify the loss ratio by operating companies or by plant location, if they had a sufficiently large employee population. Currently, we have about 150 such cost centers where we can spot overutilization if it occurs. Before this information was available, we had always looked at places like New York City, Nashville, and California. But the data from our system did not point to these places at all. The first five hospitals we identified as problems were in small communities in Tennessee and Mississippi.

At the meeting that took place in this small community in Tennessee, we carefully reviewed all the facts that we had, and then asked for the hospital's suggestions as to how we could bring utilization under control. There was absolutely no lack of candor on their part over the fact of overutilization. They blamed us for part of it owing to the way our plan was designed. They asked for reimbursement for outpatient surgery and for diagnostic care, to which we agreed and which they now have. We are waiting perhaps sixty days to see if their utilization pattern changes. If it doesn't, we will institute a certification program for this particular hospital. If that does not bring utilization under control, then we will begin refusing to pay bills from this hospital that are not medically necessary, which is a provision of our contract.

Thus, one of the results of my involvement in the health planning process has been a better understanding of how the system is affecting Genesco—what is actually happening to our health care benefits program and what we consider to be some abuses in the system.

Another thing I have learned is the sensitivity of the provider community to competitive influences. I have been involved in an advisory capacity with an ambulatory surgery center. Since this new competitive influence has come into Nashville, the hospitals have lowered their charges for outpatient surgery. In another example, the HSA recently approved an application for an HMO feasibility study. The application was emotionally attacked by the doctors. They accused the HMO of being everything from a Communist plot to an insidious plan by the federal government to implement national health insurance. What amazed me was that absolutely no one besides myself challenged these patent fallacies.

Another benefit that has accrued from my involvement in the planning process is the opportunity to disseminate ideas. At a meeting in Washington earlier this year sponsored by WBGH, I first learned about the hospice concept. Its humanitarian aspect appealed to me because terminally ill citizens are so often given no say over what happens to them during the average 3.1 months they have to live. I went back to Tennessee and learned that we had a small group in Nashville that was trying to develop this service. In checking with our Middle Tennessee HSA, I found that not only was it not in our plan but it was also totally unknown as a concept to our professional staff. We have corrected both these problems.

Finally, I have had the opportunity to share the education that has resulted from my involvement with health planning. We have developed a labor and industry advisory council, made up of only nine representatives, but, those nine people represent 200,000 consumers in middle Tennessee. This council can review and comment on all applications for certificates of need that come before the HSA. They also have opportunities to learn about things like the hospice service that is offered in Nashville.

We still have a long way to go in industry, but involvement in the health planning process is one of the best ways we can more fully understand the delivery system and influence it to the betterment of our employees and our society as a whole.

Mr. Hurst:

I am a convert, so beware of my enthusiasm. When I served in the Illinois state legislature some years ago, I voted against most governmental planning efforts. I thought they were grandiose schemes that intruded in private affairs, cost a lot of taxpayers' money, and culminated in nothing but closets full of paper. I also spent seven and a half years in labor relations negotiating with the UAW. Such matters are very specific, definable, and not plagued by the airy generalities of some planners.

From that alien background, I was dragged, kicking and screaming, onto the board of the HSA in central Illinois about three years ago. After the first year, I still had the feeling they were only churning out paper. But, when the HSA president asked me to head the HSA Plan Implementation Committee and make something happen, I agreed. My marching tune was: you planned the work—now I'll work the plan. The population in our HSA area is about 700,000. Caterpillar has about 35,000 employees in the area, so obviously, if the committee could affect the quality and cost of care, that would have a significant impact on Caterpillar.

How have we done so far in implementing our annual goals? Let's use the example of our goal to increase immunization levels. Immunization in some of our HSA region was as low as 20 percent. A state law requires grade school children to show evidence of immunization at certain grade levels, but it wasn't being enforced. I wrote to the state superintendent of public instruction asking for an explanation. He in turn sent a letter to all local school district superintendents telling them to enforce the law. The percentage of children immunized in our region has more than doubled in the last four months. Most of the credit for improvement must go to subregional task forces of citizens and organizations who volunteered under the direction and training of HSA staff to help school districts get their records in order, to help give shots, to help city-county health departments offer immunization clinics. In addition to the unquestionable benefit of fewer sick children, there is the benefit of reduced hospitalization for preventable diseases.

Another specific goal in our annual implementation plan is to reduce the number of medically underserved areas within the region. We formed a committee of several physicians, with the dean of the Peoria School of Medicine as chairman. He got together with several health departments and hospital groups and found that three or four separate groups were all pursuing doctors for the same county. They have combined their efforts and their resources, and they are going to get a doctor.

Another of our annual goals is to reduce health care costs. In theory, costs can be reduced by substituting home health care for high-cost hospitalization. Yet many employers have not provided home health care in their benefit plans. And even if they do provide the benefit, is home health care available? We formed some more task forces and found that agencies were duplicating and competing with one another, but leaving gaps in service. We got together with the agencies, and they have at least given lip service, so far, to an intent to work together toward a unified program dovetailed with the hospitals and physicians.

In Peoria, we formed a Health Services Committee of the local Chamber of Commerce. I am its chairman. Most of the major employers in the HSA region are members, as well as physicians, hospital administrators, and insurance firms. We are now in the process of education about HSAs, HMOs, PSROs, home health care, second surgical opinions, and so on. Our next step will be to ask the hospital administrators about the 1,000 or so excess beds in our HSA region. Overbedding is at least one goal that won't be resolved in twelve months, if ever.

Caterpillar has benefited directly from my involvement in health planning. In addition to the accomplishments already mentioned, through the HSA, I have become familiar with several other topical acronyms such as PSRO and HMO. We have hired the local PSRO to monitor hospital admissions and lengths of stay. This has had significant financial impact. Our average length of stay is down significantly. Also, we've expanded our examination of HMOs. We believe the HMO concept is sound, but not every execution of it is sound. We have an HMO at one of our plant locations that needs improvement. We have been dealing with its Board of Directors and administrators, pointing out specifically where we think its administration can be improved.

I encourage employees to get involved with the HSA because it seems to be the best game in town where consumers can have a meaningful impact on our health care delivery system.

Mr. Cain:

I take it as a given that we should have an effective health planning program. The question is, How do you get one?

There are clearly four essential ingredients. One is a higher level of awareness and education among the general public about the health industry and what health planning is. Two, you need adequate funding for the health planning program as it is now established. Three, you need participation from all the interests involved. Four, you need an increase in skill and sophistication on the part of the professional health planners who provide the staff services to HSAs.

There are at least two other needs that are maybe even tougher to meet. One is that Congress has to enact reasonable laws and make reasonable changes and improvements in the Health Planning Act. Two, HEW must, if it is to meet its responsibilities under the Planning Act, perform in a reasonably effective and competent way. Our association is growing largely because these last two needs aren't being met. One of the most serious challenges in the Washington arena is the set of expectations there as to what the Health Planning Program can reasonably accomplish, and when. HEW should do one of two things: either show some real competence in implementing this act, or be willing to stay out of the way. I am sorry to report that neither option is being acted on at this point. In fact, Secretary Califano has only recently expressed strong support for the Planning Program.

There are serious problems ahead in the next year. The administration worked very hard but failed to get through a hospital cost containment program, and the Health Planning Program failed to achieve a three-year extension. The great danger is that the administration may try to put the two together in the next Congress. We will probably see a renewed effort in HEW to make changes in the rules governing the selection of HSA governing boards and the interests that must be represented. Each of the proposals will seem reasonable by itself, but their combined effect may make HSAs almost impossible to run. The appropriations for this program in 1980 will probably be under very serious constraints, as will almost everything else. The rules now prohibit HSAs from accepting funds from the health insurance industry. I am anxious to explore some alternatives to total dependence on federal appropriations for the success of this program.

When the program almost came out of Congress in this past session, there were several proposed changes in it that would have seriously restricted the ability of HSAs to influence Congress or their state assemblies. In effect, these changes would have prohibited HSAs from taking public positions on controversial issues. Apart from the constitutional issue, these are particularly undesirable proposed changes because one of the principal advantages of the HSAs, when they become as effective as I think they can be, is that they will be community-based, broadly based critics of public policy in the health area.

Finally, antitrust could become a serious problem. The Justice Department apparently feels that there are antitrust issues involved in the health planning process that merit their attention.

Question Period

Willis Goldbeck, WBGH: How do HMOs fit into health planning?

Mr. Brown: I have some reservations. We have to be very careful in how we approach the pushing of HMOs because there's always a chance that you'll push a bad one. We had an HMO about three or four years ago in Nashville that stunk up the environment so much that now we cannot get people to look at HMOs in a reasonable manner.

Kevin Stokeld, Deere and Company: Deere's actual experience with HMOs began recently in Denver and Minneapolis. Although we offered the HMOs to less than 400 employees at these locations enrollment exceeded 30 percent at both units. Our most important involvement at this time is in acting as a catalyst in the Quad Cities to bring interested parties together to form an HMO. Although the closed-panel seemed more attractive at first we quickly came to the realization that the IPA model would have a better chance of fostering a positive attitude on the part of the physicians . . . And we were convinced that without such a positive attitude the HMO would be doomed to failure. We believe that cost containment and quality health care can result only from cooperation; not from coercion.

Mr. Hurst: Caterpillar has a facility in the Quad cities and is supportive of Deere's catalytic efforts. We are also involved with other HMOs. Our experience has been very good. Our data with regard to cost per employee or to the company for HMO involvement related to the company plan suggests that there is a significant dollar savings in HMOs and the quality of care is good. Out of three HMOs, we have two good experiences and one that is not so good that we are trying to fix. The health care system needs competition. HMOs are a vehicle for competition and I think we ought to support them. But we need to evaluate them on a one-by-one basis and not sell to employees a service we are not proud of.

Joan Paul, Colt Industries: I was asked to sit on an HSA but told that the final decision would be made by the person to be replaced.

Mr. Brown: That is quite different from the procedure of my HSA.

Mr. Cain: It is precisely that kind of situation that HEW will be trying to rectify with new regulations. Unfortunately, the new regulations are likely to cause as much harm as good.

William McHenry, Coopers & Lybrand: Does Caterpillar plan to extend its utilization review program? Why haven't more employers taken advantage of such programs?

Mr. Hurst: We are thinking about expansion and are currently negotiating with another PSRO. As to why more companies don't do this, not all PSROs are equally competent.

Edward Fox, Prudential: What communications, if any, had Genesco had with their employees in the area of that hospital you visited, and what was their reaction?

Mr. Brown: As we identified problem locations, we began internal reeducational programs for employees in those facilities. All our employees receive some sort of communication monthly regarding cost containment and their responsibility in the battle to contain costs under our company health care program. In the locations identified as high users, we have concentrated and tailored our programs to the specific employee groups, so they are learning, along with the providers, that we do have a problem in that community and specifically what their responsibilities are going to be in resolving that problem. If we ever get to the point where we have to stop paying claims, we will give the employees at least sixty days notice.

COMMENTARY

Daniel I. Zwick, Assistant Director, American Hospital Association

Health planning has come a long way in the United States. Still, it has a long way to go. In the next few years, we will learn whether the country has the interest and patience to develop and use this tool as an important part of the health scene. Will it receive a fair market test?

Planning in any form does not come easily in this nation. Being an activist and pragmatic people, we have usually preferred to deal with problems as they come along. This attitude has been well characterized as "act today and plan tomorrow." Similarly, communitywide planning has not been widely accepted. Experiences in such fields as land use, housing, and transportation attest to the general tendency to emphasize individual initiative and short-term solutions. Community planning has received relatively little support—and even less implementation.

In recent years, though, more people have begun to consider whether decision making might be enriched by more careful and systematic consideration of the future. This tendency has been unusually marked where research and development and long-term capital investments induce a broader perspective and a longer time frame. Discussions of planning have at least become respectable.

The health industry has many characteristics that suggest that planning might be useful. Long-term investments in facilities and professional personnel are predominant. A dollar spent today to develop a new hospital or a new physician can involve commitments that last thirty to fifty years. However,as as in other activities, planning does not come naturally to the health field. The autonomy of individual practitioners and institutions has been greatly valued. The highly personal nature of much health care has led to a reluctance to sanction excessive external interventions. Concerns for the "best" for one's own family have inclined the public to support and treasure their particular physician and hospital. The focus on individual effort and autonomy have produced substantial quality in American health care. However, it has produced many imbalances as well. As the national investment in health care increases, the imbalances have become more important and increasingly costly.

Similarly, the higher cost of health care has led to greater public interest in and some questioning of the value of certain health services. While confidence that "doctor knows best" is still common, many members of the public are willing, and even determined, to raise questions. However, the complexities and the special language of the health field has often made it difficult for "outsiders" to engage these issues effectively.

The community-based Health Planning Program, established as a result of Public Law 93–641, provides opportunities through-

out the country for those interested to engage these issues. It aims
to provide open forums for considering issues that in the past
were generally dealt with behind closed doors by medically based
boards of health and institutionally focused boards of trustees. It
seeks to bring together the wide diversity of interests concerned
with health issues to define current problems and needs to formu-
late future directions and priorities.

Community-based health planning systems are still relatively
new in this country. While earlier efforts were initiated three or
four decades ago, this type of planning has only been undertaken
seriously across the nation for ten years or so. It needs time to
develop and mature. We need to learn how to make community
health planning work. More knowledge is needed how best to
represent both consumer and provider interests. Groups that have
not traditionally interacted effectively need to learn how to act
together. More effective data and analytical approaches must be
developed and applied.

Expectations for health planning should not be unrealistically
high, therefore. Planning efforts can contribute to the development of broader understanding of health affairs and the identification of better ways of dealing with identified and anticipated
difficulties. However, they cannot alter the nature of things: they
cannot simplify things that are intrinsically complex and they
cannot create changes that do not fit the state of society. Further,
the purposes of planning should not be confused. Planning is not
decision making. While this distinction is generally clear in the
business community, it is often confused in the health field. Con-
fusion has even become more common as communitywide planning becomes more closely associated with regulatory activities,
such as capital investment and budgetary reviews.

Planners serve decision-makers; they do not replace them.
Health decision making, which has been highly fragmented in the
past, is tending to become more focused. As health care financing
delivery become more organized, the responsibilities for critical
decisions are becoming more centralized in large institutions,
multiinstitutional systems, financial agencies, and state and federal governments. Health planning can provide a framework for
better decision making. It can add perspective and purpose. However, it will not—and should not—assume the functions of the
responsible executives.

Planners are sometimes blamed for the dilemmas and difficulties they expose. Since there are important unresolved problems
in American health care, the life of the health planner can be
difficult. The search for ways to achieve "equal access to quality

health care at a reasonable cost" presents difficult conceptual and operational issues that are not likely to be solved easily or quickly in America. At its best, the planning system can help engage these complex matters in constructive ways.

If communitywide health planning is to receive a fair test of its potential contributions, two ingredients are essential. Persons interested in the improvement of health care must contribute to the consideration and formulation of community plans, and persons responsible for the management of health care must respect and help execute the plans adopted by the community. The business community has a critical role in determining whether these two ingredients are achieved and thus whether communitywide health planning will have a fair market test in America.

COMMENTARY

Scott Fleming, Senior Vice President, Kaiser Foundation Health Plan, Inc.

I approach this subject with considerable skepticism. I have characterized the health planning system, semiestablished through several rounds of federal and conforming state legislation, as "a leading example of a successful federal intervention in the health care field—a system that was designed not to work and is succeeding in not working."

On balance, the three presentations, and particularly the forthright comments of Mr. Cain on major problems with the system, did little to alter my opinion. However, lest I seem too much the cynic, let me emphasize that I was favorably impressed by the affirmative views and specific examples that Messrs. Brown and Hurst presented. I do recognize that in many parts of the country the health planning system may achieve constructive results, and I can understand why Mr. Hurst says, "Get with the HSA because it seems to be the only game in town." There may indeed be places where the health planning system is the only game in town, but I earnestly hope that business leaders such as those participating in the WBGH will not reach that conclusion until they have thoroughly explored the possibility of encouraging effective competition among alternative health care delivery systems as a potentially more effective, less expensive, and less bureaucratic means of stimulating efficiency in their local health care economies.

Mr. Brown's comments on the "sensitivity [i.e., resistance] of the provider community to competitive influences" were especially interesting. His experience supports the classic views of Adam Smith, who correctly observed that managers of enterprise generally seek to avoid, restrict, or minimize competition—quite naturally because life in a competitive field is never easy nor comfortable. Generally speaking, economic competition is viewed as fine in the abstract and good in someone else's business but not in one's own. The health care field, for professional and historical reasons, has been particularly noncompetitive (at least in traditional economic terms). Physicians regard economic competition as nonprofessional, and among traditionalists in the hospital field *competition* is a dirty word. Thus the resistance of established hospitals to an ambulatory surgery center and the resistance of physicians and hospitals to a prospective HMO are not surprising. Quite naturally, the provider community seeks to use its influence in the health planning system to inhibit potential competition. Apparently, from many reports on provider responses such as those mentioned by Mr. Brown, providers have not yet found the sultry morass of bureaucratic regulation sufficiently oppressive to make them prefer the sharp chill winds of competition.

Although I was favorably impressed by the successes that Messrs. Brown and Hurst reported within the context of their involvement in the health planning system, I was even more intrigued to note that major achievements were essentially independent of the formal health planning structure. The Nashville Ambulatory Surgery Center apparently did not require or obtain HSA approval. The Advisory Council on Health Care for Middle Tennessee represents a mobilization of labor and business influence, as a force external to the HSA, for achieving the consumer influence that HSAs supposedly incorporate.

Apparently, Mr. Hurst, experienced in both business and politics and with the support of a major company, has been remarkably effective as chairman of the HSA Plan Implementation Committee. Thus the HSA did provide the framework for his efforts, but I did not detect any achievement that *depended* on the HSA. Rather, he used factual information that the HSA staff was useful, but not essential, in developing, together with political savvy and effective business leadership.

On the really tough issue of overbedding, Mr. Hurst stimulated a Chamber of Commerce Health Services Committee as a means of mobilizing the influence of major employers, and the Tri-County Industry-Education-Labor Council which brings organized labor and the major educational institutions into the coalition. Indeed, first listening to, and then carefully reading, Mr. Hurst's presentation, I am struck by the fact that the failures of their HSA—having HSA recommendations overruled at the state or HEW level—are intrinsic features of the health planning system, whereas their successes appear to have been attainable by effective leadership and organization, and independent of the health planning system.

Advocates of the planning system will no doubt maintain that, even though much action occurs outside the formal planning structure, that structure is nonetheless an essential medium through which business, labor, and other major constituencies can influence the health care system. They will argue that the kind of constructive impacts that Messrs. Brown and Hurst reported have only become possible because of the health planning system.

I find this fallacious. Escalating health care costs have gotten the attention of business and political leadership; organized labor has recognized its community of interest with business in keeping health care costs from consuming an ever increasing portion of the wage dollar. Thus I see increased concern on the part of business, labor, and political leadership as the primary energizing factor behind the successful interventions that Messrs. Brown and Hurst reported. To credit the health planning system, as such, with these successes is no more valid than to argue: because the effort and resources put into the health planning system have increased rapidly along with the dramatic health care cost increases of recent years, therefore health planning *causes* health care cost escalation.

My comments on Mr. Cain's presentation can be quite brief. I have known Harry reasonably well as an able and conscientious public servant in HEW and in his present role as Executive Director of the American Health Planning Association—a role for which he is admirably fitted by background, experience, and sincere commitment to the health planning process. I respected his statement on his departure from HEW, which, as I recall, was substantially to the effect that he had broken his pick in a futile effort to bring HEW into effective support of the health planning system. I admire his determination and respect his optimism in trying to make health planning work from his important leadership position in the American Health Planning Association.

However, I am clearly less an optimist and more a skeptic. To the knowledgeable, critical, and thoughtful listener, Harry's presentation makes a case against the prospective effectiveness of the health planning system which, though rather different from the case I would make, is quite persuasive. He comments on possible future amendments affecting the composition of HSA governing boards and suggests that these could produce "an institution that is almost impossible to run." But aren't we there already? Among several difficult problems he attributes to the health planning system he mentions two that are "maybe even tougher"—that "Congress has to enact reasonable laws" and that "HEW has to perform in a reasonably effective and competent way" or "stay out of the way." This suggests an anecdote about the pioneer days in the Southwest. An inhabitant of that hot, dry desert remarked to a visitor about how wonderful the area was and how "all it needs is a better class of people and more water." Replied the visitor, "Why, man, that's all Hell needs."

I recognize that the southwestern states have achieved considerable success. Perhaps there is hope for the health planning system.

Industry in Community-Level Coalitions

Joseph G. Kozlowski

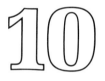

The Greater Cleveland Coalition on Health Care Cost Effectiveness is an example of an effort initiated by industry to deal with health care issues at the local level. You'll notice that is name includes the term *cost effectiveness,* not *cost containment.* We use the latter because it includes a quality improvement connotation as well. I would like to describe how this broad-based group was begun and what it plans to accomplish.

First, let me comment on why TRW got involved. Our corporate cost containment strategy says that we should be working externally as well as internally, and looking to both the short term and the long range. Examples of short-term internal activities are hypertension screening and control programs, or second surgical opinion programs, insurance modifications, benefit redesign, and HMO offerings. Internal activities, though, will not have the kind of influence that comes from working directly with the community's health system. By banding together with other groups, we can increase our leverage through shared information, additional power, and a multiplication of resources.

The coalition began at a cost containment seminar sponsored by Case Western Reserve University School of Management. All the concerned constituencies were represented—business, labor, the hospitals, the physicians, the insurers, and others. Several of us from business concurred at the meeting that getting everybody together for discussion was a positive step but only a beginning. What was needed was to move into an action phase. So we formed a cadre of people and went around the community in an effort to identify others interested in forming a coalition. It took a year to get it organized because everybody started by saying, "Yes, we're interested, but get it going first and then we'll jump in and help you."

We were finally able to get representation from all the major constituencies. Our fifteen-member Board of Directors includes two people from the insurance industry, one Blue plan person and one representing the commercial carriers, two people from business, two from labor, five providers, one person from the hospital association, one from the medical society, one representing the dentists, two representing the physician community at large, and finally, a catch-all category of four people including academics, consumers, and others.

Rather than setting up a corporation, we looked around for an umbrella organization. Of the several groups we talked to, the local HSA gave us the best offer. They provided a mailing address, stationery, stenographic assistance, and a telephone answering service, all with no strings attached. These were all helpful since we are a voluntary effort.

Having found a base of operations, we proceeded to write a constitution. In retrospect, I think we should have done that sooner, since it helped to clarify our objectives and could have been useful in convincing people to join. We put together a board and elected officers. As the last part of our organizational phase, we sketched out five broad issues on which we might fruitfully put task forces to work. They are: data base and health economics, health education, provider efficiency, optimum hospital capacity, and incentives to cost effectiveness and optimal utilization.

We've just completed the organizational phase, and we are starting the action phase. Among our first objectives is to increase the community's level of awareness of our existence and the issues giving rise to it. Right now we are drafting a press release and designing a booklet to convey some information about who we are, our overall goals, and what we're trying to do. Our statement of goals is cast in general terms, and we think it covers the range of possibilities and likely solutions.

From our experience I can offer a few words of advice for others who want to form a similar group. First, think in terms of a long-term commitment. A community organization is not the kind of thing that you can handle in six months or a year. Second, involve all the constituencies. I have seen some groups focus on business exclusively and, at the local level, I consider that a mistake. Third, try to find a central theme to focus your initial efforts. Our inclination right now is to spend our first year of activity on building awareness throughout the community. Finally, don't let yourselves be coopted by anyone. Make sure that you remain business-oriented and don't get pulled into long, academic studies.

Question Period:

Ronald Hurst, Caterpillar Tractor: Why did the coalition not use the Chamber of Commerce as the umbrella organization?

Mr. Kozlowski: The problem with the chamber is that they have their own bureaucracy, and any time we wanted to take a position we would have to clear it through them. Keeping it voluntary and independent gives us more flexibility. As a matter of fact, though, the chamber has been very helpful to us.

John Prescott, American Can: What would be the disadvantage of restricting such a group to business people?

Mr. Kozlowski: Ultimately, it is going to be the physicians and the hospitals who change the health care delivery systems—and I deliberately use the plural. We as business can best act as a catalyst to get them working on cost containment and quality improvement. We can do a lot of internal things independently, but we can't really change the system without their participation.

William McHenry, Coopers & Lybrand: How can the coalition keep from being coopted given that only four members of the board represent business and labor?

Mr. Kozlowski: No one dominates the board. It was deliberately structured in such a way that there's a balance of power, even though it sounds like there are a lot of provider representatives. Interestingly, it's the insurance carriers who tend to be the swing votes.

Arthur Lifson, Equitable Life: Could you address the question of funding?

Mr. Kozlowski: The coalition is going through a formal membership campaign right now. Part of this is to find out who's really committed, so we're asking for dues of $100 from organizations and $25 from individuals. Till now, it has been a totally voluntary effort, with organizations donating occasional space or helping with various costs. We don't intend to raise any large sum of money, though. If we get to a point where we need monies to fund specific studies, we plan to seek foundation support.

Edward Fox, Prudential: Has the coalition begun any activities to reduce overbedding in the Cleveland area?

Mr. Kozlowski: We have not been in existence long enough to have had an impact. Our energies so far have been devoted to establishing credibility with organizations like the hospital association. This means convincing them, for example, that we are not a bunch of madmen out to close every hospital in the community. It's taken a long time to establish that credibility, and we are really just beginning to move into the action phase.

COMMENTARY

Ronald A. Hurst, Manager Health Care Planning, Caterpillar Tractor, and Member, Central Illinois Health Systems Agency

Many of Mr. Kozlowski's experiences and suggestions are useful and applicable at most locations. For example, his matrix of company activities that are either long-term or short-term and either internally or externally directed is valid for most places and most organizations. He also concentrated on the need for initiative and the necessity for follow-through. He pointed out the desirable leverage in group activities and the usefulness of a neutral forum such as a university. He also appropriately mentioned involving the HSA and providing publicity to enhance public awareness of the health care problem.

However, I would offer this specific caution: the activities of any company need to be tailored to the nature of that company and its locale. For example, the activities of a company with large concentrations of employees in a few areas can differ significantly from those of a company with many scattered but small establishments. Obviously, it should be simpler for an organization with a large concentration of employees in a single area to effect changes (remembering, of course, the danger of a high profile while implementing changes that may not be welcomed or understood).

Second, the chamber of commerce may be the most appropriate vehicle in other places. In some locales, such as our own in Peoria, the chamber can be one of several effective forums that obviate the need for establishing another new organization such as the Cleveland Coalition. In fact, I chair a new committee of the Peoria Chamber of Commerce called Health Services. Our purpose is to educate the major employers in the area as well as the medical establishment and insurance companies regarding the nature of the health care cost problem. Once there appears to be understanding of HSAs, HMOs, PSROs, the lack of competition, and so on, we will begin to look at possible actions to solve the problem. While it is true there is no labor representation on the Chamber of Commerce committee, there is another organization in this area called the Tri-county Industry-Education-Labor Council which is active and effective. I intend to involve that organization for the same purposes of education and action. Fortunately, Bradley University is located in Peoria and can provide a neutral forum or catalyst if that proves appropriate.

There also exists in the Peoria area a Central Illinois Industrial Association which is an umbrella for major manufacturers. Here and elsewhere, the HSA is well-organized and well-staffed and will be of use. My point in referring to these organizations is to emphasize that it may not be necessary to form a new organization. If there are good ones presently operating, my suggestion is to involve them rather than to form a new group. Obviously, this avoids duplication or dilution of efforts.

Mr. Kozlowski did not refer to HMOs or PSROs in his presentation. Since we have both in our area, I am also weaving them into the education/action activities generated by the organizations mentioned above. For example, the directors of the PSRO and HMO will speak at one of our upcoming Chamber of Commerce meetings to describe their groups and will undoubtedly get new subscribers after the presentations. The same applies to our HSA director.

Finally, I think the following quotation from *The Prince*, by Machiavelli, way back in 1513, is quite relevant to America's current health care delivery problems:

> It must be considered that there is nothing more difficult to carry out, nor more doubtful of success, nor more dangerous to handle, than to initiate a new order of things. For the reformer has enemies in all those who profit by the old order, and only lukewarm defenders in all those who would profit by the new order; this lukewarmness arising partly from fear of their adversaries, who have the laws in their favour, and partly from the incredulity of mankind, who do not truly believe in anything new until they have had actual experience of it. Thus it arises that on every opportunity for attacking the reformer, his opponents do so with the zeal of partisans; the others only defend him half-heartedly, so that between them he runs great danger.

THE CHALLENGE
REVISITED

Industry as Change Agent

Richard H. Egdahl, M.D.

At this conference, we've heard a strong case for increased government involvement, a larger role for the insurance companies, and negotiated fees for doctors—plus, limitations of total health spending. This is a viewpoint that we as providers have to take cognizance of. Years ago, it wouldn't have mattered much because there wasn't any move to contain costs. Speaking now as a provider—a surgeon who is also responsible for a hospital—I must say that we have been given a fair degree of latitude to get our house in order in the private sector. If that doesn't happen, with industry's assistance to the HMO movement, to the Voluntary Effort, and so on, then there will be further government involvement. Perhaps the nationalization, in effect, of this one industry whose costs some feel are totally out of line might be accepted by the industrial world. The providers must realize that it's an alternative.

New forces, particularly industry, have been drawn into the health care decision-making arena by rising costs. We all support the VE, but we must recognize that there are some basic problems with it. I would like to pinpoint the areas that we should focus on now to help make the VE work and help preserve the private health care system. I will briefly bring up five points which have not received much attention so far at this conference.

Medical Technology

The first centers around technology and technology assessment. Much of the discussion so far about hospital cost containment has not made clear that some portion of hospital cost increases is due to new technology. And, as the industries developing the new products well know, they are not necessarily aimed at increasing cost efficiency, but more often toward improvements in accuracy or effectiveness of instruments, devices, or systems. For instance, our lab group has been working for years with Joslin Laboratories in Boston on the development of an artificial beta cell. This is a small but complex device that will ultimately be implanted in diabetic patients to normalize their blood sugar. Many diabetologists think it will prevent many of the complications of diabetes. We can predict that a lot of people are going to want that device, but it will be extremely costly. What does cost effectiveness mean here? Certainly, at least in the short range, costs will be greater.

This is just one example of many such technologies being developed. My terrible concern is that, although I am fully supportive of the VE, we're going to have to make some tough decisions on the new technology. We may have to ration it somehow by only paying for new technology that "works," or the VE has no long-range chance of success.

A lot of people in the government are already working on technology assessment—among them Seymour Perry in NIH, Dave Banta in the Office of Technology Assessment in Congress, Gil Omenn in the Office of Science and Technology in the White House, and Clif Gaus with Health Care Financing. These offices and others may get together and work out some demonstration experiments before certain new procedures are put into the reimbursement formulas—something that wasn't done with the coronary artery by-pass procedure. The private sector, with much money involved in prototype development and possible future sales and yet so much other money in employee health benefits packages, may want to express an informed viewpoint on new technology and technology assessment.

There are some built-in conflicts. Some of these products will be cost ineffective, perhaps, if you look at just one life versus many.

Industry ought to get together and make some value judgments, just as it does on national health insurance and HMOs, because technology assessment is going to be a very big issue over the next several years with Congress and the administration. That dialogue is one that industry must be part of, because it ultimately will determine a share of health care costs.

Medical Research

A second issue that I've heard not a word about, and that I think is equally important, is biomedical research. We have entered a new era in research where priorities are being set. I am not talking about re-search evaluation—our present peer review system for evaluating research, basic and clinical, works very well. Rather, I'm talking about Secretary Califano's recent challenge to the National Institutes of Health to focus on the the hard questions of priority and choice in order to provide guidelines to indicate the type of research that should be supported. The secretary stressed that NIH should emphasize the relationship between health research and unmet health needs and encourage a dialogue among the nation's laboratories, the health care delivery system, and the regulatory process.

I submit that industry must be part of this dialogue. Research priorities have previously been largely decided by the political process. A strong and articulate group would get a lot of money for this or that type of research. But now it's being said in HEW that they are going to set five- and ten- and fifteen-year goals for the relative allocation of research dollars. Now, if there is any relationship between the allocation of those dollars and the relative importance to society of the diseases being studied, and if that has to do with health care cost premiums—and I think it does—then an informed group of industrial people should have an input to that process, along with other consumers, providers, researchers, and regulators. This is quite an indirect approach to health care cost control, I admit, but nobody is now looking for a quick fix. One way we might hope to bring costs down eventually is to assess and rank our general targets for research, just as we do in many of the other areas under discussion.

This is going to be a big battlefield, because every special interest group with this or that disease in mind will apply pressure. But what industry can do is come at it as empirically as possible. Industry already funds much research, including very basic research, through contributions committees or through collaboration with universities. There hasn't been much involvement previously with the public policy issue of the general direction of biomedical research, but public research monies have reached the stage where groups other than research societies are looking at priorities. Industry should be in on that process, whatever it is.

Physician Issues

My third point concerns physicians—how many, what kinds, and what they charge. One of the vital policy issues due to be thrashed out in the next few years is whether we are training too many doctors. Being a physician with responsibility for a medical school, I am protective in this situation; but some feel that we are training too many physicians, and the way that medical schools are supported is increasingly becoming an issue in the public eye.

A second part of the manpower problem centers around the ratio of specialists to primary care providers. This also partly reflects the way medical education is funded, and it sometimes presents problems of access to consumers. I know of places that are saturated with specialists, but primary care doctors are not to be found.

Finally, we have fees. The medical establishment makes a strong argument for controlling fees within the profession, but there are very strong forces developing that want to participate in the decision. Some say fees are too high and should be brought into line with state or federal fee schedules. Also, there are certain anomalies in fee structures. For example, we see much higher surgical fees in some large urban areas, where there is often an oversupply of surgeons, than in some less populated areas where surgeons are needed. Some countries, Canada for instance, have set fee levels at least partially to achieve appropriate geographical distribution.

I am not suggesting what industry's position should be on the issues of number of doctors, ratios of specialists, and whether fee schedules are developed at a state or national level. However, for industry not to be involved in the dialogue when it has accelerated to the national level and is being actively discussed by HEW and congressional committees constitutes a denial of its active role in cost containment.

Long-Term Care Facilities

My fourth point concerns long-term care facilities and programs. One of the frustrations in running a hospital is that we may get charged for medically unnecessary days when there is no appropriate place to send the patient. Adequate long-term facilities don't exist in many parts of this country, and yet one regulatory group says, "If you don't get our patients out when they no longer have to stay in the hospital, you won't get paid for the hospitalization, even if there is no one to take care of them at home." If you don't have ways to get people out of very costly acute-care facilities into more appropriate long-term care facilities, it will cripple cost containment efforts and, in some cases, even hamper correct treatment.

The lack of long-term care facilities is a bottleneck that will plague us for many years to come. As long as we don't have adequate ways to care for patients who do not need to be in the hospital but are not ready to go home, we will continue to have excess inpatient days. I make the plea that industry look carefully at this issue and adopt a stance on it.

Utilization Review and Control

My final point concerns the use of claims data to actually do utilization review. Many companies say they're already doing that, but not too many really have a program for using claims data for controlling overutilization. You probably don't need to contemplate utilization review if your area has competing prepaid health plans, including a closed-panel HMO, an IPA, and an unstructured fee-for-service system that will be under the pressure of price competition.

If you don't have competing plans, you're stuck. Your only hope to keep health care costs in line is vigorous claims review. You need three things to make it work. First, the corporations and the carriers, or, if corporations are self-funded, whoever's managing the claims, have to agree on exactly what data are needed and what to do with them. Most big insurance companies pay claims fast and accurately, but they don't routinely compile the extra data necessary to do utilization review. You have to have an agreement that you're going to get the infornation and specify what you need. Second, you need to have models for diagnosis and treatment performance standards defined by physician advisers. If the local PSRO is taut and effective in peer review, then you hire it. But that may not be true in all instances, and if it isn't, then you have to do it yourself with your own physician-advisers.

Third, you computerize the information, array it, and analyze it. You may find some "black hats"—providers who are doing very strange things like giving vitamin B_{12} shots several times a week—but there's not really much savings there because most physicians attempt to practice high-quality medicine. The real savings occur in cutting down one day of hospitalization or decreasing the use of unneeded lab tests—that sort of thing. Making this happen takes a strategy, somebody who will send letters to the doctors (holding the patient harmless financially), letters to the hospital the day of admission, saying: "This is your length of stay. Beyond it we won't pay." There is some preliminary evidence that this kind of utilization review of claims data may have a payoff.

In addition, third-party utilization review of this sort may provide same kind of stimulus to the fee-for-service system that a closed-panel HMO would. The Minneapolis fee-for-service plan that we've heard about here included precertification—if the doctor doesn't get the admission approved in advance, the bill doesn't get paid. With this kind of rigor, the doctors had to change their practice patterns, and they initially didn't like it. Why did they accept it? There were six closed-panel plans taking away their business at a fairly rapid rate. So they clamped down on hospital overutilization. Unfortunately, you aren't going to find the Minneapolis phenomenon existing everywhere, so a third-party utilization control program is an alternative. If you're located in an area that's hopeless in terms of having competitive pre-paid plans, then look at your claims, develop standards for diagnostic and treatment procedures, and begin to institute some activities that have some potential for cost containment.

I've outlined five specific areas that members of the WBGH should become knowledgeable about and become involved in over the next few years. The success of the VE and the future of the private health care delivery system, if there is one, depend very much on finding solutions to these problems, among others.

Question Period

James Tobin, Becton-Dickinson: I'm concerned about lumping technology like the beta cell diabetes control unit into the problem of cost containment. Shouldn't we measure cost-benefit and cost containment on different tracks?

Dr. Egdahl: That's a question that we agonize over all the time. The beta cell will be something like renal dialysis or a transplant: it will cost a lot and huge numbers of people will want it. Unless it's going to be at the expense of something else, then we'll have to accept it as an add-on to health care cost inflation. Some say maybe we ought to do just that, whereas others look at the bottom line and say we have to make a decision. I think the beta cell is like the coronary by-pass. It may well be useful for one category of patient but not for another, and a value judgment has to be made. The real question is whether we are just going to start using it or are we going to have some kind of outcomes validation and public debate before it becomes automatically fitted into the reimbursement equation? This is an ethical question *and* dollars-and-cents question, too. Industry should be thinking about it and making an informed input to the debate about the inclusion of new procedures in the reimbursement formula. Industry has the resources to do some selected cost-benefit studies.

John Virts, Eli Lilly: It seems to me that a second reason, besides cost control, for doing the claims review you suggest is simply to determine whether our benefit programs are working the way we expect them to with the people who really need them, and also to find out whether there is something about the work environment or the community environment or whatever that is causing particular health problems. We can actually improve the total system with a management-by-exception sort of utilization review, not just control costs.

Philip Lescohier, William M. Mercer: What relative value do you attach to precertification of hospital admissions as compared with concurrent in-hospital review as a means of controlling hospital utilization?

Dr. Egdahl: You get variable responses from different places around the country. The data aren't hard, as you know, but precertification was the thing that seemed in Minneapolis to turn things around. Precertification adds a certain something extra, and it makes the physician and the patient come to grips with whether the admission is essential.

Q.: Has anybody done any real microanalysis of health care costs to see where increases are originating—how much is new technology, how much is increased utilization, how much is inflation, and so on?

Dr. Egdahl: All of us in the field have looked for studies of the sort you describe and they are hard to find. I'm not sure that the microeconomic approach is productive given the current status of the data, but certainly, we have some outstanding health economists who are becoming deeply involved in this area. The trouble is, as we've found in our studies on the performance of fee-for-service HMOs, the further you dig in the data, the less satisfying the data are.

Appendix

Conference Participants Quoted
"1978 Annual Meeting of the Washington
Business Group on Health"
Washington, D.C.: October 30–31, 1978

George N. Bates, M.D., Medical Director, Owens-Illinois, Inc., Toledo,
Ohio
John Brown, Director, Employee Benefits, Genesco, Inc., Nashville,
Tennessee
W. Gordon Binns, Jr., Assistant Treasurer, General Motors Corporation,
New York, New York
Harry P. Cain, Jr., Executive Director, American Health Planning As-
sociation, Alexandria, Virginia
Irvine H. Dearnley, Vice President, Citibank, New York, New York
H. Peter deLisser, Director, Health Programs, The Executive Health
Examiners Group, New York, New York
Henry A. DiPrete, Second Vice President, John Hancock Mutual Life
Insurance Company, Boston, Massachusetts
Winfield C. Dunn, Senior Vice President, Public Affairs, Hospital Cor-
poration of America, Nashville, Tennessee

Paul W. Earle, Executive Director, The Voluntary Effort, Chicago, Illinois

Richard H. Egdahl, M.D., Director, Boston University Center for Industry and Health Care, Boston, Massachusetts

Marion Ein, Associate Director, National Health Policy Forum, Washington, D.C.

Paul M. Ellwood, Jr., M.D., President, InterStudy, Excelsior, Minnesota

Richard E. Emrick, Manager, Benefit Programs, Mead Corporation, Dayton, Ohio

Jonathan E. Fielding, M.D., Former Commissioner of Public Health, Commonwealth of Massachusetts, Boston, Massachusetts

Max W. Fine, Executive Director, Committee for National Health Insurance, Washington, D.C.

Edward W. Fox, Senior Consultant, Health Policy Coordination, Prudential Insurance Company of America, Newark, New Jersey

Cramer M. Gilmore II, Assistant Director of Research and Education, International Brotherhood of the Teamsters Union, Washington, D.C.

Willis B. Goldbeck, Director, Washington Business Group on Health, Washington, D.C.

Clark C. Havighurst J.D., Professor of Law, Duke University; Adjunct Scholar in Law and Health Policy, American Enterprise Institute; Consultant, Federal Trade Commission, on antitrust in health care, Durham, North Carolina, Washington, D.C.

Lawrence C. Horowitz, M.D., Staff Director, Subcommittee on Health and Scientific Research, Washington, D.C.

Robert C. Hendrickson, Corporate Director, Employee Benefits, The Sherwin-Williams Company, Cleveland, Ohio

Samuel H. Howard, Vice President Planning, Hospital Affiliates International, Inc. Nashville, Tennessee

Ronald A. Hurst, Manager, Health Care Planning, Caterpillar Tractor Company, Peoria, Illinois

Stanley B. Jones, Program Development Officer, Institute of Medicine, Washington, D.C. (formerly Professional Staff Member, Senate Subcommittee on Health)

Ronald H. Kilgren, Employee Insurance Department, Ford Motor Company, Dearborn, Michigan

H. Peter Kneen, Jr., Director, Employee Benefits, IBM Corporation, Armonk, New York

Joseph G. Kozlowski, Corporate Manager, Employee Benefits, TRW, Inc., Cleveland, Ohio

Philip R. Lescohier, Consultant, William M. Mercer, Inc., Chicago, Illinois (formerly Manager, Employee Insurance, International Harvester)

Lawrence S. Lewin, President, Lewin and Associates, Inc., Washington, D.C.

Arthur Lifson, Senior Association, Health Affairs, Equitable Life Assurance Society of the United States, New York, New York

Freddie H. Lucas, Industry-Government Relations, General Motors Corporation, Washington, D.C.

J. Michael McGinnis, M.D., Deputy Assistant Secretary for Health (Disease Prevention and Health Promotion), Department of Health, Education, and Welfare, Washington, D.C.

William P. McHenry, Jr., Coopers and Lybrand, Washington, D.C.

David F. McIntire, Manager, Employee Benefits, General Mills, Inc., Minneapolis, Minnesota

Judith K. Miller, General Director, National Health Policy Forum, Washington, D.C.

Kenneth J. Morrissey, Manager, Employee Benefits, FMC Corporation, Chicago, Illinois

Neils H. Nielsen, Director, Personnel Services, ARA Services, Inc., Philadelphia, Pennsylvania

Joseph N. Onek, Associate Director, Domestic Policy Staff, The White House, Washington, D.C.

Jan Peter Ozga, Associate Director for Health Care, U.S. Chamber of Commerce, Washington, D.C.

Joan Pastor, Director, Employee Benefits, Colt Industries, New York, New York

John E. Prescott, Manager, Benefits Planning and Special Projects, American Can Company, Greenwich, Connecticut

Mike A. Riley, Director, American Medical Association, Washington, D.C.

John J. Salmon, Counsel, Subcommittee on Select Revenue Measures, Committee on Ways & Means, U.S. House of Representatives, Washington, D.C.

Bert Seidman, Director, Department of Social Security, AFL-CIO, Washington, D.C.

Bruce D. Sidebotham, Director, Employee Services, General Tire and Rubber Company, Akron, Ohio

Michael W. Soulier, Manager, Employee Benefits Section, E.I. DuPont de Nemours, Wilmington, Delaware

Kevin M. Stokeld, Manager Health Care, John Deere and Company, Moline, Illinois

Donald E. Strange, Director of Research, The Center for Health Studies, Nashville, Tennessee

James R. Tobin, Director of Public Affairs, Becton-Dickenson and Company, Paramus, New Jersey

Nila A. Vehar, Staff Coordinator, Government Affairs, Koppers Company, Inc., Pittsburgh, Pennsylvania

Howard R. Veit, Director, Office of Health Maintenance Organizations, Washington, D.C.

John R. Virts, Ph.D., Corporate Staff Economist, Eli Lilly and Company, Indianapolis, Indiana

Diana Chapman Walsh, Associate Editor, Springer Series on Industry and Health Care, Boston University Center for Industry and Health Care, Boston, Massachusetts

M. Keith Weikel, Vice President, American Medical International, Washington, D.C.

Kenneth W. White, Vice President and General Manager, Health Insurance Institute, Washington, D.C.

Daniel I. Zwick, Assistant Director, American Hospital Association, Washington, D.C.